Women in Pediatrics

Nancy D. Spector • Jennifer K. O'Toole
Barbara Overholser
Editors

Women in Pediatrics

The Past, Present and Future

Springer

Editors
Nancy D. Spector
Executive Leadership in Academic Medicine® (ELAM), Office of Faculty
Drexel University College of Medicine
Philadelphia, PA
USA

Barbara Overholser
Drexel University College of Medicine
Executive Leadership in Academic Medicine® (ELAM), Philadelphia, PA
USA

Jennifer K. O'Toole
Internal Medicine-Pediatrics Residency Program, Departments of Internal Medicine and Pediatrics, University of Cincinnati College of Medicine, Cincinnati Children's Hospital Medical Center
Cincinnati, OH
USA

ISBN 978-3-030-98221-8 ISBN 978-3-030-98222-5 (eBook)
https://doi.org/10.1007/978-3-030-98222-5

This Springer imprint is published by the registered company Springer Nature Switzerland AG
The registered company address is: Gewerbestrasse 11, 6330 Cham, Switzerland

We dedicate this book to the women in pediatrics and medicine that have gone before us. We stand upon their shoulders as we strive to achieve equity and advancement for all women.

We also dedicate this book to the generations of women in pediatrics and medicine that will follow us. We sincerely hope that they will encounter a very different experience in their careers. We hope they will have the opportunity to practice in an environment where they feel truly valued, supported, and elevated, and have access to fully equitable and safe workplaces.

Foreword

The first quarter of the twenty-first century has seen the status of women in medicine and pediatrics improve slowly, even if by fits and starts, only to suffer a significant negative impact caused by the ongoing COVID-19 pandemic.

In many professional environments, attitudes and behaviors identified as positive in men are looked askance and rejected if exhibited by women. While women comprise a vastly larger number of residents and practicing pediatricians than men in the USA, there are significantly fewer women pediatricians than pediatricians who are men in leadership positions such as chairs of departments. Still now, there is a noticeably diminished presence of women physicians on boards of hospital and healthcare systems, with women taking a preferentially supporting and nurturing role in undergraduate and graduate medical education, as well as part-time employment to better care for their families.

Recent data indicate that, over a lifetime of employment, women physicians earn on average up to $2 million less over the course of their career than their counterparts who are men [3]. Women have traditionally faced decreased compensation, and delays in promotion and achievement of upper-level leadership in academic medicine.

Programs specifically designed to advance leadership skill acquisition in women, such as the Executive Leadership in Academic Medicine Program® (ELAM), have significantly contributed to help improve the status of women physicians in leadership roles. Much work, however, is still needed especially as the recent COVID-19 pandemic has placed a disproportionate burden of family care and job-related stress on women physicians, negatively impacting their careers [1, 2].

The editors and authors of this book are uniquely qualified to raise a voice and examine the disparities hitherto in place in the workplace. They clearly explain the impact of intersectionality on equity and the inordinate toll that gender discrimination has on the wellness and opportunities of women in pediatrics, which mirror those of women in medicine in general.

This book delves into the historical antecedents of the challenges affecting women in pediatrics today and presents the readers with viewpoints often stemming from the authors' own personal journeys, reflecting the fact that many of the challenges of yesteryear continue to be mirrored today. The authors distinctly delineate with clear, certifiable, and trustworthy data historical inequities that demand repair and resolution.

More importantly, perhaps, this book constructs a positive blueprint for a brighter and more equitable future, aimed at correcting inequalities, supporting women pediatricians (and women in general) in their career development by understanding the dynamic circumstances, and developing an environment of promotion and allyship.

This book tells us that we still owe our women colleagues nothing more and nothing less than equity.

Daniel V. Schidlow
Dean Emeritus, Professor of Pediatrics Medicine
Pharmacology and Physiology Formerly Physician in
Chief, St. Christopher's Hospital for Children and Chair
Department of Pediatrics, Drexel University College of Medicine
Philadelphia, PA, USA

References

1. Jagsi R, Fuentes-Afflick E, Higginbotham E. Promoting equity for women in medicine – seizing a disruptive opportunity. N Engl J Med. 2021;384(24), 2265–67. https://doi.org/10.1056/NEJMp2104228.
2. Weiner S. How COVID-19 threatens the careers of women in medicine. 2020. Retrieved July 24, 2021 from https://www.aamc.org/news-insights/how-covid-19-threatens-careers-women-medicine.
3. Whaley CM, Koo T, Arora VM, Ganguli I, Gross N, Jena AB. Female physicians earn an estimated $2 million less than male physicians over a simulated 40-year career. Health Affairs. 2021;40(12):1856–64. https://doi.org/10.1377/hlthaff.2021.00461.

Preface

We were approached to write this book in late 2019 following the publication of *Women in Pediatrics: Progress, Barriers, and Opportunities for Equity, Diversity, and Inclusion* [7]. That manuscript detailed the challenges and barriers women in pediatrics face despite making up the majority of the specialty's workforce and also proposed a system by which gate keeper groups could help eliminate those barriers. However, that paper was written prior to the COVID-19 pandemic, and since that time, priorities have shifted and evolved. The initial effect of the pandemic on women in medicine has been substantial, and the long-lasting impact has the potential to set women in medicine back by decades. There is no better time than right now to tell the story of women in medicine, highlight the struggles and discrimination they face, and truly hold organizations and leaders accountable for leading meaningful change.

The story of women in pediatrics is unique and incredibly valuable. Pediatrics is a specialty in which women compose almost two thirds of the workforce. Unlike other specialties, we have overcome the challenge of getting women into the specialty; however, women are still suffering from the impact of gender segregation and systematic sexism within the specialty [5]. This has resulted in fewer women obtaining leadership roles, delayed advancement, salary inequity, burnout, job dissatisfaction, mental health disorders, and attrition. Not only are women battling the effects gender segregation in pediatrics, they also face isolation from other more senior women in the specialty (e.g., the "queen bee" phenomenon resulting from a gender-biased environment) and the "pediatrician stigma" in which they are "too nice" and falsely believed to be poorly equipped to assume high-powered leadership roles. This "triple threat" puts women in an extremely precarious position and is likely amplified in specialties outside of pediatrics.

While sharing the story of women in pediatrics may be of great value to the larger medical community, it is important to recognize that we are just one small piece of the puzzle, representing less than 10% of the total physician workforce in the USA [1]. Therefore, leaders in the field of pediatrics must align with leaders in other specialties to ensure efforts to help all women in medicine are working collaboratively and united under a central purpose. We must not exist in a silo, and it is our moral imperative to swiftly share our learnings and progress with other specialties to benefit all women.

While this book is about *women* in pediatrics, we hope that *all in medicine* will read and learn from this book regardless of their gender identity. We speak now specifically to men in our field. In holding the majority of the positions of power and influence, your acknowledgment of the bias and systemic sexism women face and your engagement in efforts to create change are critical. Women cannot do this alone. They need your support, your allyship, and your sponsorship. You are the ones that can create true change and help fashion a workplace that truly values, supports, elevates, and provides an equitable workplace for women in the field.

We hope this book not only shares the past and present story of women in pediatrics but also inspires all of us to create a world where all women in pediatrics and in medicine can thrive. Pediatrics is in a very unique position to change the course of history and create that world. If a specialty that is predominantly women and prides itself in supporting women as mothers and caregivers cannot achieve this goal, who can? In a post-pandemic world, this work is more important than ever, and pediatrics must lead the way and create a standard for the rest of medicine to follow.

Philadelphia, PA, USA — Nancy D. Spector
Cincinnati, OH, USA — Jennifer K. O'Toole
Philadelphia, PA, USA — Barbara Overholser

References

1. AAMC Physician Specialty Data Report: Active Physicians in the Largest Specialties, 2019. Retrieved July 14, 2021 from https://www.aamc.org/data-reports/workforce/interactive-data/active-physicians-largest-specialties-2017
2. ADVANCE PHM. Retrieved December 20, 2021 from www.advancephm.org.
3. American Women's Medical Association. Retrieved August 9, 2021 from https://www.amwa-doc.org/.
4. Executive Leadership in Academic Medicine program. Retrieved October 7, 2021 from https://drexel.edu/medicine/academics/womens-health-and-leadership/elam/.
5. Pelley E, Carne M. When a specialty becomes "women's work": trends in and implications of specialty gender segregation in medicine. Acad Med. 2020;95(10):1499–506. https://doi.org/10.1097/ACM.0000000000003555.
6. Promoting and Respecting our Women Doctors – PROWD. Retrieved December 20, 2021 from https://twitter.com/prowdwomen.
7. Spector ND, Asante PA, Marcelin JR, Poorman JA, Larson AR, Salles A, Silver JK. Women in pediatrics: progress, barriers, and opportunities for equity, diversity, and inclusion. Pediatrics. 2019;144(5). https://doi.org/10.1542/peds.2019-2149.

Acknowledgments

Women in Pediatrics: The Past, Present and Future would not have been possible without the extraordinary efforts of its chapter authors. We are grateful for their contributions to the book, to the field of pediatrics, and to promoting gender equity in medicine. We'd also thank the Legacy Center Archives and Special Collections at Drexel University College of Medicine and its archivists, Matt Herbison and Kieran McGhee, for their research assistance and access to the fascinating stories of early pediatricians. We'd also like to thank our colleagues at Executive Leadership in Academic Medicine® (ELAM), ADVANCE PHM, the American Medical Women's Association (AMWA), and Julie Silver, MD, and Promoting and Respecting our Women Doctors (PROWD). It will take a coordinated effort among advocates to achieve the goal of gender equity in medicine, and we are grateful to collaborate with these exemplary organizations. We're also thankful to our own mentors, sponsors, and allies.

Contents

Contributors

Sharon Calaman Department of Pediatrics, Division of Pediatric Critical Care, New York University Grossman School of Medicine, New York, NY, USA

Douglas Carlson Department of Pediatrics, Southern Illinois University School of Medicine, HSHS St. John's Children's Hospital, Springfield, IL, USA

Archana Chatterjee Rosalind Franklin University of Medicine and Science, Chicago Medical School, North Chicago, IL, USA

Tina L. Cheng Department of Pediatrics, University of Cincinnati, Cincinnati Children's Hospital Medical Center, Cincinnati Children's Research Foundation, Cincinnati, OH, USA

Eliza Lo Chin American Medical Women's Association, Schaumburg, IL, USA

Laura Chamorro Dauer University of Miami Miller School of Medicine, Miami, FL, USA

Louito Edje University of Cincinnati Medical Center, Cincinnati, OH, USA

Catherine Forster UPMC Children's Hospital of Pittsburgh, University of Pittsburgh, Pittsburgh, PA, USA

Jorge F. Ganem PeaceHealth, Abigail Ln Eugene, OR, USA

Alda Maria Gonzaga University of Pittsburgh School of Medicine, Pittsburgh, PA, USA

Rita P. Guevara Drexel University College of Medicine, Philadelphia, PA, USA

Yemisi Jones Continuing Medical Education, Hospital Medicine, Cincinnati Children's Hospital Medical Center, Cincinnati, OH, USA

Anika Kumar Cleveland Clinic Lerner College of Medicine of Case Western Reserve University, Cleveland, OH, USA

Kheyandra D. Lewis Drexel University College of Medicine/St. Christopher's Hospital for Children, Philadelphia, PA, USA

Howard Yee Liu UNMC Department Psychiatry, UNMC COM, Nebraska Medical Center, Omaha, NE, USA

Kelsey Logan Division of Sports Medicine, Cincinnati Children's Hospital Medical Center, University of Cincinnati College of Medicine, Cincinnati, OH, USA

Vineeta Mittal Department of Pediatrics, UTSW Medical Center & Children's Health, Dallas, TX, USA

Kayce Morton Jordan Valley Community Health Center, Cox Health, Springfield, MO, USA

Jennifer K. O'Toole Internal Medicine-Pediatrics Residency Program, Departments of Internal Medicine and Pediatrics, University of Cincinnati College of Medicine, Cincinnati Children's Hospital Medical Center, Cincinnati, OH, USA

Mary Ottolini Tufts University School of Medicine and The George W. Hallett MD Chair of Pediatrics, The Barbara Bush Children's Hospital at Maine Medical Center, Portland, ME, USA

Barbara Overholser Executive Leadership in Academic Medicine® (ELAM), Drexel University College of Medicine, Philadelphia, PA, USA

Shilpa J. Patel Pediatrics at University of Hawaii, John A. Burns School of Medicine, Pediatric Hospitalist at Kapiolani Medical Center for Women & Children, Hawaii Pacific Health, Honolulu, HI, USA

Glenn Rosenbluth University of California, San Francisco, San Francisco, CA, USA

Samir Shah Division of Hospital Medicine, Cincinnati Children's Hospital Medical Center, Cincinnati, OH, USA

Department of Pediatrics, University of Cincinnati College of Medicine, Cincinnati, OH, USA

Eleanor Sharp UPMC Children's Hospital of Pittsburgh, University of Pittsburgh, Pittsburgh, PA, USA

Erin E. Shaughnessy Department of Pediatrics, University of Alabama at Birmingham, Birmingham, AL, USA

Pam Shaw University of Kansas School of Medicine, Kansas City, KS, USA

Nancy D. Spector Executive Leadership in Academic Medicine® (ELAM), Office of Faculty, Drexel University College of Medicine, Philadelphia, PA, USA

Amy Starmer Department of Pediatrics, Boston Children's Hospital, Harvard Medical School, Boston, MA, USA

Beth A. Tarini Center for Translational Research, Children's National Research Institute, Children's National Hospital, The George Washington University, Society for Pediatric Research, Silver Spring, MD, USA

Anisha Thaker University of Massachusetts, Amherst, MA, USA

Teri L. Turner Baylor College of Medicine/Texas Children's Hospital, Houston, TX, USA

Karen M. Wilson Department of Pediatrics and the Clinical and Translational Sciences Institute, University of Rochester School of Medicine, Rochester, NY, USA

Part I
Where We Started – History of Women in Pediatrics

Chapter 1
Stories of Early Leaders/Early Days of Women in Pediatrics

Barbara Overholser, Jennifer K. O'Toole, and Nancy D. Spector

Introduction

Pediatrics is considered a more recent specialty within the timeline of medicine. Long before Abraham Jacobi and Job Lewis Smith, the men considered to be founders of the specialty in the mid-nineteenth century, the needs of infants and children were supported by families, friends, and midwives, but rarely physicians [16]. Concurrently, Elizabeth Blackwell, M.D., the first woman to be admitted to and graduate from a US medical school in 1849, opened a dispensary in New York City in 1857 to provide focused care for poor women and children. But it wasn't until the late nineteenth century that the importance of medical care of children was recognized by established medicine, and perhaps only because it was brought forth by men. In 1880, Abraham Jacobi and other physicians founded the American Medical Association's section on the diseases of children, and 8 years later, their new organization, the American Pediatric Society, helped to sanction pediatrics as a definitive area of medicine [15].

B. Overholser
Drexel University College of Medicine, Executive Leadership in Academic Medicine® (ELAM), Philadelphia, PA, USA
e-mail: Bro29@drexel.edu

J. K. O'Toole (✉)
Internal Medicine-Pediatrics Residency Program, Departments of Internal Medicine and Pediatrics, University of Cincinnati College of Medicine, Cincinnati Children's Hospital Medical Center, Cincinnati, OH, USA
e-mail: jennifer.otoole@cchmc.org

N. D. Spector
Executive Leadership in Academic Medicine® (ELAM), Office of Faculty, Drexel University College of Medicine, Philadelphia, PA, USA
e-mail: Nds24@drexel.edu

N. D. Spector et al. (eds.), *Women in Pediatrics*,
https://doi.org/10.1007/978-3-030-98222-5_1

As the field of pediatrics grew, and as more women entered medicine in general, women physicians seemed to find a more viable home in this specialty than in other areas. "While women were not generally accepted in medicine, their role in pediatrics was more acceptable to men, who essentially controlled medicine" [7]. Now, 64% of active pediatricians are women [1].

There are countless interesting and important stories of the accomplishments of women in pediatrics that could be shared for this chapter. We chose to highlight three women who practiced during different eras and had varied life experiences. They each deserve recognition for their roles in the historic timeline of the field and for the inspiring lives they led.

Mary Putnam Jacobi, M.D. (1842–1906)

Mary Corinna Putnam was born into the Putnam publishing family of New York on August 31, 1842. She graduated from the Female Medical College of Pennsylvania, the first medical school in the world for women, in 1864, the only student in the history of the school to write her thesis in Latin [17]. But even though a medical school for women existed in the USA, opportunities for women to obtain additional medical education and training were still extremely limited. Dr. Putnam left for Paris, France, where she spent 5 years studying medicine and science, including time in microbiology labs, studying histology and cellular pathology. She was the first woman admitted to the l'Ecole de Médecine and received the highest mark for a thesis, graduating with a second M.D. degree in 1871:

> "Miss Putnam," says a Paris paper, "the young American who has for some years been following the course in l'Ecole de Médecine, submitted her graduating thesis to the Faculty. It was read in the large lecture room of the College before a numerous audience, and was received with warm commendation. The President of the Board of Examiners found it deserving of the highest note-'extrémement satisfait.' This mark is rarely given for a thesis. Miss Putnam has also received the highest mark at each of her five Examinations. She writes that one of the dedications of her thesis was as follows: 'To the professor, whose name I do not know, who alone voted in favor of my admission to the Ecole, thus protesting against the prejudice that would exclude women from superior studies." [14]

Dr. Putnam returned to New York City in 1871 and opened an office in her father's house. In 1873, she and Dr. Anne A. Angel began to attend to children brought to the Mount Sinai Hospital dispensary, establishing the pediatric service at the hospital [14]. She later opened a children's ward at the New York Infirmary in 1886. While her new husband, Abraham Jacobi, would go on to be called the "father of pediatrics," Mary Putnam Jacobi built her own reputation as an educator, practitioner, and leader at various medical institutions in New York City (Fig. 1.1).

She used science to prove that "women were biologically capable of being equal players in the public sphere" [2]. From the earliest days, women physicians have had to contend with fear-based resistance from colleagues who were men who "worried that female physicians would degrade the profession with their poor

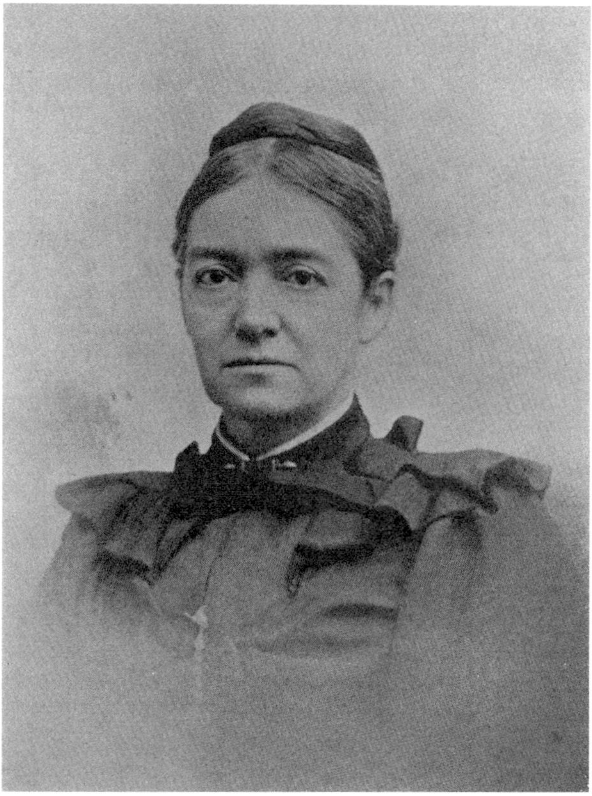

Fig. 1.1 Mary Putnam Jacobi, undated, item number p0066a. Legacy Center Archives, Drexel University College of Medicine, Philadelphia

training and frail constitutions" [2]. But within that backdrop, Mary Putnam Jacobi was able to gain a national and international reputation for her knowledge, skill, and tenacity, thus transcending that resistance, at least in some respects. "Medical men held her in high regard, seeing her as an exceptional woman of talent and genius" [2]. Dr. Jacobi wanted to see women fully integrated into the field of medicine. "She deplored the tendency of women doctors 'to nestle within a little circle of personal friends and to accept their dictum as the ultimate law of things'" [17].

In 1872, Dr. Jacobi organized the Association for the Advancement of the Medical Education of Women which later became the Women's Medical Association of New York City. She served as its president for almost 30 years [4]. Dr. Jacobi became the first woman fellow of New York Academy of Medicine in 1880.

Outside of medicine, she was a published author and a suffragist, and the address that she presented on women's suffrage to the New York State Constitutional Convention of 1894 in Albany is cited as an important contribution to the subject [18]. *"Common Sense" Applied to Woman Suffrage* is an expanded form of that address, and in the introduction by Frances Maule Björkman in the book's second edition, we see the significance of Dr. Jacobi's contribution to the suffragist movement. "The bringing of Dr. Jacobi into active relationship with the organized suffrage movement was a distinct triumph, for the reason that she brought to the cause not only a personal and family prestige of great value, but the best of all qualifications—the practical demonstration in her own career of woman's capacity in untried fields" [13].

Martha May Eliot, M.D. (1891–1978)

Dr. Martha May Eliot was a pediatrician, policymaker, and humanitarian who devoted her career to the health and well-being of women and children, both as a practitioner and as an advocate. She graduated from Radcliffe in 1913, applied to Harvard Medical School which did not admit women, and instead attended Johns Hopkins School of Medicine where she received her medical degree in 1918. She graduated with her classmate Ethel Collins Dunham who would become her life partner [3]. She and Dunham, who was also a pediatrician, were devoted to each other and built their personal and professional lives around each other, coordinating opportunities when they could. "While Dunham and Eliot are each worthy of individual attention, their shared personal life has such an intimate connection with their careers that a combined narrative better illustrates their close relationship of 59 years. They achieved major professional positions at Yale, at Harvard, and in government, even while they were making careful career choices to maintain the continuity of their domestic partnership" [10].

In 1921, Eliot became the first women resident physician at the New Haven Hospital. She became a protégé of the pediatrician Dr. Edwards A. Park, and together they published definitive work on rickets, establishing the importance of early diagnosis and developing an economical cure that included daily requirements for vitamins [6, 10]. She taught in the department of pediatrics at Yale until 1934, and while at Yale, she was appointed director of the US Children's Bureau's Division of Child and Maternal Health in 1924. Ten years later, she became the Bureau's assistant chief, while her partner Dunham became chief in 1935. Eliot was appointed head of the Children's Bureau in 1951 where she continued to influence maternal and child health policy. "For Dr. Eliot, the Children's Bureau was a base for her to carry out her professional role as a women physician as well as the traditions of the women reformers and the previous female chiefs of the bureau" [19] (Fig. 1.2).

In her resignation letter from the Bureau, Eliot wrote of the need to prioritize the health of children:

> Those of us who are engaged in work for children are keenly aware, however, that much needs to be done. Far too many children fail to benefit from the advances that medicine, education and the biological and social sciences are constantly making. Our goal is the optimum development of every child. If this is to be attained, the needs of children must receive much higher priority in our public and personal budgeting of time, thought, and money, than they now receive. In my mind, there is no more important matter before us today. [8]

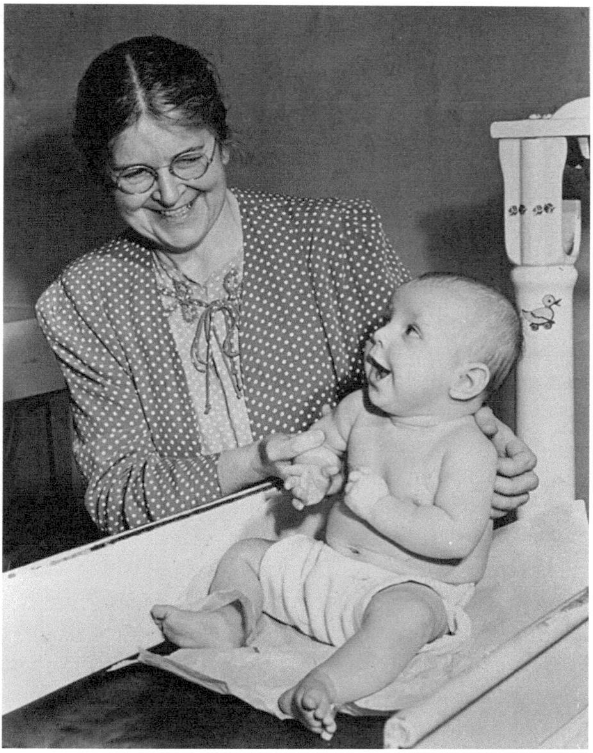

Fig. 1.2 Dr. Martha May Eliot holding and weighing an infant on a scale. 1951. Schlesinger Library, Harvard Radcliffe Institute

Dr. Eliot had many "firsts" including being the first woman president of the American Public Health Association, the only woman to sign the originating document of the World Health Organization, and the first woman awarded the American Public Health Association's Sedgwick Memorial Medal. She and Dunham were the first two women admitted to the American Pediatric Society. Eliot's work with the Emergency Maternity and Infant Care program, a wartime government program that was "the nation's largest maternal and infant care operation, providing medical and hospital care to nearly a million and a half wives and infants of servicemen in the four lowest pay grades" [6], earned her a Lasker Award in 1948, making her the second woman Lasker awardee.But while she led an extraordinarily successful and prominent professional life, she was still subject to discrimination based on her gender and sexuality. Both she and Dunham were attacked by Senator James Reed of Missouri in a tirade against the Children's Bureau in 1921, when he called the bureau out as a place where 'the only people capable of caring for babies and mothers of babies are ladies who have never had babies' [12].

Eliot's obituary in *The New York Times* did not mention her long partnership with Dunham, referring to her only as "Dr. Martha May Eliot, an unmarried woman who devoted her life to problems of maternity and child care" [20].

Roselyn Payne Epps, M.D., M.P.H. (1930–2014)

Roselyn Payne was born in the segregated south of Little Rock, AK, on December 11, 1930, and devoted her career to promoting the health of children and women. Both of her parents were educators—her father, Dr. William K. Payne, Sr., was president of Savannah State College (GA), and her mother Mattie Beverly Payne was a counselor in the Savannah, GA, public schools. It was at the age of 10 that she declared that she wanted to be a pediatrician. "I was interested in a career that linked children, scientific inquiry, and helping others" [5]. She attended Palmer Memorial Institute, a college preparatory school that was founded by a Black woman physician and graduated at 16. She received her undergraduate and medical degrees from Howard University (she was one of eight women in her class, about 10% of the class) and completed her rotating internship and pediatric residency at Freedmen's Hospital where she served as chief resident. She later received an MPH from Johns Hopkins School of Public Health and Hygiene and a Master's degree in Interdisciplinary Studies from American University in Washington, DC.

Dr. Epps' career spanned the gamut and included time as a practitioner, a researcher, an administrator, and as a visiting scientist at the National Cancer Institute of the National Institutes of Health. She had a 20-year career with the District of Columbia's Department of Public Health and held positions including Pediatric Medical Officer and Director of the Clinic for Retarded Children. Dr. Epps was a Professor of Pediatrics and Child Health at Howard University and also the founding Director of the High-Risk Young People's Project, Chief of the Child Development Division, and Director of the Child Development Center at the university. As director of the Howard University Child Development Center, she brought together physicians, community service organizations, and members of the private sector to establish a community-based facility to treat people ages 15–24. The Child Development Center was described as an "international force in pediatric health issues and preventative medical care for elementary school children" and was extremely important to the residents of Washington, DC, neighborhoods [11]:

> I grew up in the segregated South, on the campus of Savannah State College in Georgia. So in a way I was insulated. When I applied to medical school, I realized things might be different than what I had known. When I went around to medical school interviews I was asked "Why don't you just get married and have children? When was in medical school and during my internship, sexism and racism were there, though there are no particular incidents that stand out. Sometimes there were sexist jokes or statements. I was one of eight women in my medical school class. When I was asked to join a local chapter of the American Medical Women's Association, half of the white members resigned. Maybe I should have quit, but the ones who left were the ones with the problems. [5] (Fig. 1.3)

Dr. Epps was the first African American and first woman to become president of the District of Columbia Chapter of the American Academy of Pediatrics. Outside of medicine, she was involved in numerous organizations and became the national president of Girls Inc. where she sought to expand the organizations' cultural programs. "(I) think it's important to have these cultural programs. If a girl has confidence in herself, she can face anything in her environment" [9].

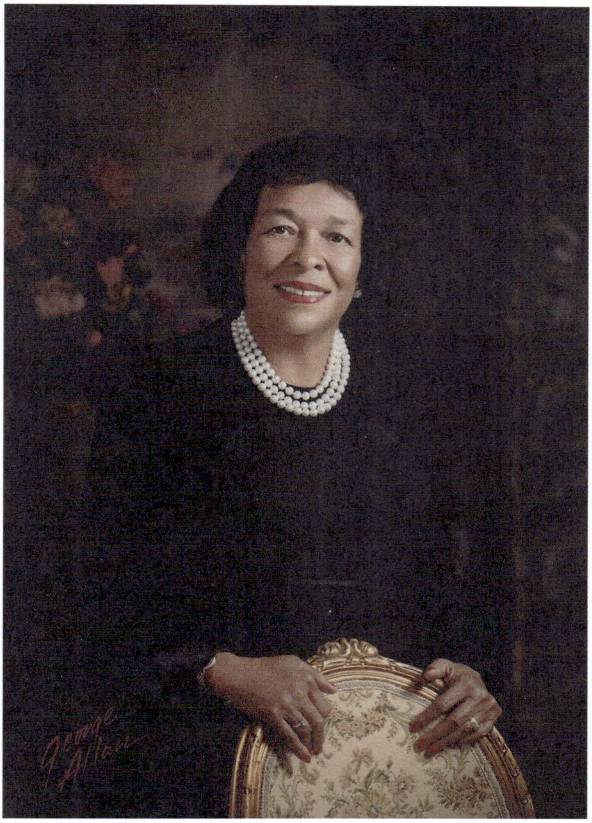

Fig. 1.3 Roselyn Payne Epps, M.D., M.P.H. Photograph by George Allan. (Courtesy of Charles H. Epps, Jr., M.D., and Roselyn E. Epps, M.D.)

Dr. Epps was intensively involved with the American Medical Women's Association (AMWA). She was the first African American to serve as president and received the organization's highest honor—the Elizabeth Blackwell Award. In collaboration with AMWA, she co-edited *The Women's Complete Healthbook*, a landmark 700-page medical reference text.

In her AMWA inaugural address as president on November 3, 1990, in Philadelphia, Dr. Epps said: "The future of medicine will depend on the full participation of women physicians in setting the policies and agenda for medicine. ...Even as we serve as mentors for those who are entering our noble profession – and I do believe it is noble – we must reach down to young girls considering their career choices."

Dr. Epps recognized the importance of mentorship in her life, acknowledging the roles her working mother and her high school principal had in instilling determination and values [5]. And she saw an important role in "paying it forward" by helping the women who came after her in the field of medicine. "I have been able to help other women in medicine—to open doors, hold them open, and help women through. I have enjoyed being a mentor to others. My approach is to always look at what I can contribute and do to advance something" [5].

Her deep and important contributions in the community were succinctly recognized in Constance Battle, MD's letter nominating Dr. Epps for AMWA's Community Service Award. The work of Dr. Epps, she said, "stands as a model for all physicians who desire to enrich the community in which they live."

While we were only able to share vignettes of the lives of these three extraordinary women pediatricians, we can see a common thread—that women have been instrumental in shaping the field of pediatrics while contending with significant challenges along the way. The perseverance required of these three physicians was remarkable and set the stage for future women to enter the field. Because of them and others, pediatrics went from being a field that wasn't recognized at all to becoming what is now a core field of medicine. But women in pediatrics still face many challenges, and as we commented in the Preface, even with women being the majority of physicians in pediatrics, they are in the minority of pediatric leaders. And on top of facing the challenges that are unique to women, they also face the stigma of pediatrics being considered on a lower rung of medical specialties, thus perpetuating salary inequity and impacting the field's influence in medicine in general. And this lack of influence is costly in terms of the health and well-being of the world's most vulnerable and least vocal population—children. Fortunately, the future looks bright for women in pediatrics, and we look forward to the next chapter in our history.

References

1. Active Physicians by Sex and Specialty, 2019. n.d. AAMC. Retrieved November 22, 2021, from https://www.aamc.org/data-reports/workforce/interactive-data/active-physicians-sex-and-specialty-2019.
2. Bittel C. Mary Putnam Jacobi and the politics of medicine in nineteenth-century American. Chapel Hill: University of North Carolina Press; 2009.
3. Changing the Face of Medicine | Martha May Eliot. n.d.. Retrieved November 23, 2021, from https://cfmedicine.nlm.nih.gov/physicians/biography_99.html.
4. Changing the Face of Medicine | Mary Corinna Putnam Jacobi. n.d.. Retrieved November 22, 2021, from https://cfmedicine.nlm.nih.gov/physicians/biography_163.html.
5. Changing the Face of Medicine | Roselyn Payne Epps. n.d.. Retrieved November 23, 2021, from https://cfmedicine.nlm.nih.gov/physicians/biography_102.html.
6. Davis LM. Her job is world health. Med Womans J. 1949;939;41–42
7. DeAngelis C. Women in Pediatrics. JAMA Pediatr. 2015;169(2):106. https://doi.org/10.1001/jamapediatrics.2014.2917.
8. Eliot MM. Resignation Letter. Drexel University; 1956, October 31.
9. Hampton N. Girls Inc. Chief Wants to Empower Little Women. *The Washington Times*. 1990, August 2.
10. Hansen B. Public careers and private sexuality: some gay and lesbian lives in the history of medicine and public health. Am J Public Health. 2002;92(1):36–44. https://doi.org/10.2105/AJPH.92.1.36.
11. Healing America's Children. Black Enterprise Magazine, 84. 1988, October.
12. Ilacqua, J. Pride Month Collection Highlight: Ethel Collins Dunham and Martha May Eliot. History of Public Health at Harvard. 2018. https://guides.library.harvard.edu/public-health/LGBTQ.

13. Jacobi MP. "Common sense" applied to woman suffrage; a statement of the reasons which justify the demand to extend the suffrage to women, with consideration of the arguments against such enfranchisement, and with special reference to the issues presented to the New York state convention of 1894, 2nd ed. New York: G.P. Putnam's Sons; 1915.
14. Jacobi MP. Mary Putnam Jacobi, M. D., a pathfinder in medicine, with selections from her writings and a complete bibliography edited by the Women's Medical Association of New York City. New York: G. P. Putnam's sons; 1925.
15. Late-Nineteenth and Early-Twentieth Century Pediatrics • Nursing, History, and Health Care • Penn Nursing. n.d. Retrieved November 22, 2021, from https://www.nursing.upenn.edu/nhhc/home-care/late-nineteenth-and-early-century-pediatrics/.
16. Mahnke CB. The growth and development of a specialty: the history of Pediatrics. Clin Pediatr. 2000;39(12):705–14. https://doi.org/10.1177/000992280003901204.
17. Morantz RM. Feminism, professionalism, and germs: the thought of Mary Putnam Jacobi and Elizabeth Blackwell. Am Q. 1982;34(5):459–78. https://doi.org/10.2307/2712640.
18. Putnam R. Life and letters of Mary Putnam Jacobi. New York: G. P. Putnam's sons; 1925.
19. Terrell MH. "Some kind of social doctor": historical study of Martha May Eliot's policies for maternal and child health [Brandeis University]. 1990. https://www.proquest.com/docview/303883421?accountid=10559.
20. Treaster JB. Martha Eliot. The New York Times. 1978, February 23. https://www.nytimes.com/1978/02/23/archives/martha-eliot-worked-in-child-care-use-of-social-workers-award-in.html.

Part II
Current State of Affairs

Chapter 2
Women Entering Pediatrics

Kheyandra D. Lewis and Teri L. Turner

Introduction: What Do You Want to Be When You Grow Up?

> *When I was young, I was often asked, 'What do you want to be when you grow up?' I would emphatically state, 'I want to be a doctor like my mommy!' Now that I am being inducted into the honor society Alpha Omega Alpha, I wish my mother would have had the same opportunities to be recognized as a medical student and eventual pediatrician, that I now have. We've come a long way in gender equity but we're not there yet. – Reflection by a Pediatric Trainee*

Girls no longer all want to be princesses and ballerinas; a nationwide survey of 500 children between the ages of 1 and 10 years of age conducted in 2015 revealed the most popular profession for girls was the wish to be a doctor [28]. This same survey found more girls, 41%, want to go into science, technology, engineering, and math careers than boys, at 32% [28]. A longitudinal study by the Organisation for Economic Co-operation and Development found a shift from teachers to doctors in top occupation choice cited by girls from 2000 to 2018 [64]. The future is becoming brighter for women entering the field of medicine.

K. D. Lewis (✉)
Drexel University College of Medicine/St. Christopher's Hospital for Children, Philadelphia, PA, USA
e-mail: KDL62@drexel.edu

T. L. Turner
Baylor College of Medicine/Texas Children's Hospital, Houston, TX, USA
e-mail: tturner@bcm.edu

N. D. Spector et al. (eds.), *Women in Pediatrics*,
https://doi.org/10.1007/978-3-030-98222-5_2

Setting the Landscape: Medical Student Journey

Four years – that's the length of time it takes to graduate from medical school. By the end of a medical student's third year, they embark on an individualized path to the type of physician they will be. Years before the acceptance letter is received, many know exactly what type of physician they will become. Several factors may redirect or affirm that decision: lifestyle, previous personal experience, or financial means. No matter the factors, the "fit" is often influenced by an individual or group of individuals in the desired role to which one aspires to attain.

It is not an easy journey. Each student can account for a myriad of challenges that may have had them reconsider the long hours at some point in their training. For women students in particular, the challenges are magnified with gender disparities and inequities. Women accounted for more than half of all medical students for the first time in history in 2019 and the number continues to increase [1, 7, 10, 11]. Despite the rising number, only 45.8% of residents and fellows in ACGME-accredited programs are women [11]. As the journey continues for women, representation dwindles. Despite the increasing number of physicians that are women, there are only approximately 36.3% women as practicing physicians [11]. It is imperative that these students have selected advisors and mentors to guide and impart recommendations on how to succeed. Unlike other medical specialties, pediatrics is uniquely positioned to influence the development of other women physicians as it is comprised of about 64.3% of women [11].

Influence: The Role of Mentoring

> *It is well known that women do not network as well as men and have more difficulty identifying career mentors and finding mentoring opportunities, thus ensuring significant disadvantage for academic advancement.* ([90], p. 1003)

The landscape of networking looks very different for men and women across careers. The informal "old boys' club" classic descriptor of networking emphasizes the opportunity to interchange business and friendship, accounting for larger social circles and the likelihood of greater opportunity toward career advancement for men [13]. Conversely, women often enter networking with a focus on "building long-term personal connections" [13] with a foundation of trust which inevitably creates a smaller pool of reliable confidants, and ultimately a limited reach. It has been detailed throughout the literature that women who have the guidance of a mentor are more likely to be promoted to professor than those who do not [90]. Universally, medical schools have established women in medicine committees and offices to support ongoing mentorship and address such topics as gender bias. [See Chap. 12 for more on mentorship.]

The Imposter Syndrome

In spite of their high achievement, women are more likely to experience imposter syndrome, "the internalized fear of being fraudulent despite evidence indicating success," ([38], p. 1508) which additionally contributes to lack of feeling like one belongs. It only takes a few steps down the hallway of a typical medical school before the portraits that adorn the walls remind a woman that it was not all that long ago when she in fact did not belong [38]. Although this book is focused on women in pediatrics, the path to pediatrics requires that a student, no matter their gender, must demonstrate knowledge and skill within other fields of medicine. While rotations will vary from institution to institution and individual experience, it is far too common for a woman to question her position through the journey. Fellowship and camaraderie aid in the sense of belonging and value; and these relationships are cemented in commonalities. In a study by Babaria et al. [5], women students throughout their third-year clerkships were asked to discuss their experiences. Many detailed that while on rotations they were more likely to form relationships with ancillary staff or nurses that were also women while their counterparts formed relationships with attendings who were more often men. Those same women students recognized that the differences in these relationships placed them at a disadvantage. One such student stated: "I think the outcome of this is going to be that the relationships and bonds that I've formed in this year are going to be very much, ones of—where I feel like I'm supporting female interns and nurses, and that the males in my class are going to come out with a lot of powerful relationships with people who are going to write them recommendations for future powerful positions … it's kind of important … And it's really shown me, this past month, how easy it is to get ahead when you're a man. It's not that I didn't know that already, it's just made it more clear (Surgery)" ([5], p. 862).

Distinct Qualities and Personality Traits of a Pediatrician

> *There is a common belief that women's nature makes them inherently more suitable for certain work regardless of their demonstratable skills or experience [Webb, 1997].* ([68], p. 484)

Women are three times more likely than men to choose pediatrics as a specialty [83]. In 2020, almost 4000 women medical students applied to pediatric residency [1]. Characteristically, most people would say that pediatricians are nice. In fact, a qualitative study in England interviewed women who identified that they chose the field of pediatrics because of the "nicer" work environment with colleagues, both men and women, viewed as "more supportive and approachable" [68]. The field of pediatrics innately cultivates a nurturing environment, as the role of a pediatrician is to care for not only the patient but also the patient's family. The partnership that develops between a pediatrician and a patient's caregiver is unlike any other within the medical field: a simultaneous challenge and privilege to share in the experience of the family as a whole. This team approach in care often requires longer conversations and understanding of caregiver goals. Various studies have discussed skills and characteristics of women as compared to men, such as expression of empathy, inquiry and listening style, and teamwork dynamics that impact the way in which they may select a career [47]. This alignment of values found in pediatrics and the attributes commonly portrayed by women may enhance overall career satisfaction.

There are certainly commonalities with personality types and attributes of those within the field of medicine as many choose this career to help and heal others. Women, being described as nurturing, are not unique to medicine, nor are stereotypical designations that imply a soft or docile demeanor. Unfortunately, such stereotypical descriptors are often utilized in the evaluation of women students as their standout quality and less emphasis is placed on describing their competence or knowledge.

In a study by Axelson et al. [3], women medical students were more likely to be described as "sensitive," "enthusiastic," and "compassionate" as compared to men who were more often to be described with regard to their intellect as a "quick learner" [3]. No matter the adjectives or descriptors used, we've seen in numerous studies that women often excel in care delivery. It has been shown that women physicians universally "provide preventative care more often, utilize more patient-centered communication, and provide more psychosocial counseling" to their patients than men [85].

Work-Life Integration: Impact of Societal Expectations on Women Entering Pediatrics

"I bet you would have been a much better trainee if you would have taken more time off to stay at home with your new baby than coming back after 6 weeks." – Statement made by a man to a woman colleague when she overheard him at the residency rank meeting state that a woman medical student should be ranked lower because she just had a baby. (Anonymous, 2017)

In 2020, 100 years after the 19th amendment was ratified and women got the right to vote, the Pew Research Center conducted a survey of 3143 US adults to understand Americans' views of the current state of gender equality [49]. Of those who said the USA had not gone far enough in giving women equal rights to men, differing societal expectations and family responsibilities were two of the top five obstacles noted. The American College of Obstetricians and Gynecologists states: "A woman's peak reproductive years are between the late teens and late 20s. By age 30, fertility (the ability to get pregnant) starts to decline" [41]. This is also the same timeline that women physicians are going to college, finishing medical school, and then entering 3 years of pediatric residency training. Taking time off for maternal leave during any portion of this continuum can delay graduation from one stage to the next in our time rigid training environment. Not only can it delay graduation but women who do have children during training face demanding work hours, limited options for parental leave and child support, and potential stigmatization by peers and supervisors [21]. Although overt discrimination toward physician mothers has decreased, implicit bias toward physicians who are women with children remains [29]. Chapter 7, "Childbearing, Adoption, Motherhood, and Eldercare by Women in Pediatrics," discusses motherhood and childbearing more in detail.

Career choice is influenced by personal needs and family circumstances. Often there is a challenge to meeting the responsibilities of family and the demands of career. Women hold a societal role as mother and organizer of the household and as caregiver for an elderly parent, child, spouse, or other relative [90]. Although men are capable of and fill similar roles, the default is for women to sacrifice working productivity to tend to household duties, also known as the "second shift" [45]. Unfortunately, women continue to face work-family conflict more so than their male counterparts [46]. The number of couples – two physician partners – entering the Match has tripled from 347 in 1987 to 1224 in 2021 [63]. Having both individuals in a household going through residency training at the same time places an additional burden on both these individuals due to the limited time to assist in day-to-day actions necessary to maintain a household and/or to tend to childcare duties.

> *About 1890, Sir William Osler is reputed to have written to a young (male) doctor about to marry: 'A doctor needs a woman who will look after his house and rear his children: a Martha whose care will be for the home.'*
>
> *In 1971, a McGill medical student aptly expressed her sentiments about this issue: 'I doubt if there would be as many really successful women doctors as men-unless, that is, women, as well as men, were entitled to that key of male success, a wife. By a wife, I mean someone who will wash floors, vacuum, prepare meals, wash socks, and look after our babies, all without demanding a penny in wages, someone who will take calls from our patients and type and proofread our important journal articles, and books, and someone who will invest all his or her energies in giving us the emotional sustenance we need to keep going through a full day of teaching, rounds, patients and evening committee meetings. Only when the institution of wifehood in its present form is either abolished or made available to doctors of both sexes will women physicians be able to do as much as their male colleagues'.* ([66], p. 340)

Applying to Pediatrics: What Makes a "Good" Pediatric Trainee

> *Student Doctor X is caring and compassionate in her interactions with her patients, is a hard worker and is a wonderful teacher to her peers. – Wording in a Letter of Recommendation for a woman medical student applying for pediatric residency*

Each year, pediatric residency training programs seek to find the best medical students to fulfill the program's mission. Students applying to pediatric programs submit an application packet which includes letters of recommendation (LORs), the

Medical Student Performance Evaluation (MSPE), US Medical Licensing Exam (USMLE) scores, a personal statement, and a curriculum vitae outlining experiences in medical school and college. Programs select candidates to interview who they feel will be successful in their program based on the information in the application packet. Gender differences of both the applicant and the reviewer can impact the outcomes of this selection process.

Letters of Recommendations (LORs)

Research has demonstrated gender biases in letters of recommendation in several medical specialties [30, 36, 48, 59, 60, 84, 86]. Although data is lacking in pediatrics, LORs written for applicants who are men were determined to be more "authentic" and contained significantly more references to drive, power, and work constructs compared to letters written about a woman applicant [30, 60]. Women tend to be described using grindstone characteristics such as "committed," "tireless," and "hardworking" [84] and with words emphasizing communal characteristics of teamwork, helpfulness, and compassion [59]. LORs often provide a narrative description of applicants' noncognitive traits. It is not the traits themselves that are either good or bad, but instead it is the perceptions of the individual making the assessment of whether or not these traits make a 'good physician.'

Medical Student Performance Evaluations (MSPEs)

Based on societal gender norms, women are expected to use "communal" language and engage in collaborative behaviors, avoid self-promotion, and not use aggressive/assertive language. Linguistic gender norms have also been noted in MSPEs [75]. Women medical students in this study were statistically more often described using the words "bright," "organized," "caring," "empathetic," and "compassionate" compared to their counterparts who were men [75]. However, there were no significant differences in standout words (i.e., exceptional, outstanding, excellent) [75]. The authors suggest by incorporating holistic, narrative descriptions of applicants that possible implicit biases may undermine the Deans' objectivity.

Clerkship performance is another area within the MSPE where gender may impact the chances of a women matching in pediatrics. Gender has not been found to be an independent predictor of core clerkship grades [14]. However, other studies have demonstrated that women scored higher than men on various domains of clinical performance or on examinations, yet despite these higher scores in clinical or assessment performance, there was no difference in the final grade [18, 27]. There were also gender-based linguistic differences in clerkship narrative comments as we have discussed with LORs [27].

Personal Statements

Studies have demonstrated that when women fail to adhere to gender stereotypes, they are penalized [25, 42, 43, 69, 78]. Researchers demonstrated when women trainees behaved counter to the gender-based norm, they felt they needed to apologize for being authoritative [55]. But what about the women-dominated field of pediatrics? Do gender norms remain the same when students write their own personal statement for applying to the field? Both women and men used communal language equally, but men did use agentic language of reward significantly more than their women counterparts [4]. These researchers suggest residency applicants may be subjected to dual pressures of demonstrating they belong (i.e., "fit") in the field, while at the same time uphold linguistic gender norms. Indeed, previous research from the men-dominated medical fields demonstrated that women tended to stay within the confines of social norms by writing more often about communal and social themes compared to men, although both equally used self-promoting language [23, 72, 73]. Women applicants also had more references to women in their personal statements which suggests the importance of women mentoring and role modeling in men-dominated fields [23].

Experiences in Medical School

The research is mixed when reviewing other aspects of the medical school application packet. Despite the real-life conversation above, there was no statistical difference noted in the likelihood of being inducted into AOA between men and women medical students with the same clerkship grades [89]. Women as a whole, however, were statistically more likely to be inducted into the Gold Humanism Honor Society which the authors postulated is due to the society's stated criteria of selected individuals who demonstrate empathy and patient-centered care (compassion and communal words). In a separate study, differences among the genders were also noted on the US Licensing Exam. Men outperformed women on Step 1, but this was reversed on Step 2 and there were no differences on Step 3 [77]. Gender-specific data is lacking on women specifically going into pediatrics. Personal correspondence from one of the largest pediatric training programs which receives over 1600 applications annually (approximately one-third of all 4000 annual applications) revealed gender differences in some areas which are opposite to the research data if all women regardless of specialty were included (M. A. Ward, MD, personal communication, April 15, 2021). The average number of publications was greater for men than women (6.6 vs. 5.7, $p = 0.04$), men had fewer volunteer experiences compared to women (8.8 vs. 10.5, $p < 0.01$), and men scored slightly lower in this sample than women on USMLE Step 1 (227 vs. 229, $p = 0.04$). There were no statistical gender differences in the number of students who were inducted into Alpha

Omega Alpha or the Gold Humanism Honor Society, nor in work or research experiences.

Gender differences were also noted in the literature for who volunteered to become small group leaders during the first year of medical school [88]. Both men and women view men as being more capable leaders [24, 44, 76, 79]. Medical students who were men were more likely to volunteer for emergent leadership positions by being a small group leader than women [88]. However, this gap was eliminated when the genders were equally divided among the groups (compared to self-selection of groups) and when additional instructions to bolster "belonging" were included. Therefore, how a task is described may help overcome stereotype threat.

Clinical Learning Environment: Experiences of Trainees

> *"I had a woman colleague in medical school who reported one of her supervising physicians for unwanted sexual advancements. She was forever labeled as a 'troublemaker' and I decided thereafter that there were only negative consequences for reporting. And the person she reported didn't even get into any trouble. So why should I report?" (author's (TLT) experience)*

Mistreatment of Women Along the Continuum of Medical Education

Bullying, discrimination, and sexual harassment of women trainees are far too common in the clinical learning environment [16, 17, 32, 39, 57]. A survey of senior students from 14 different US medical schools found that 69% of women had experienced gender discrimination and sexual harassment (GD/SH), twice as frequently as men [71]. Most of these experiences occurred in the clinical versus the preclinical environment, and the clinical supervising physician was the most frequent source of the behavior [32]. Women perceived GD/SH significantly more in specialties with higher numbers of men [71].

Despite efforts to eradicate mistreatment, women medical students experienced greater sexual harassment over time and not less [35], and these experiences continue as they transition to residency [37, 40, 50, 52]. The vast majority of bullying and GD/SH go unreported [19, 20, 40, 51, 58, 61]. Trainees in the GME environment rarely reported mistreatment and statistically less often than the medical students [40]. The three most common reasons for not reporting were a perception that the incident was not important enough, nothing would be done about it, and fear of reprisal. These negative experiences have significant short- and long-term consequences including decreased ability to learn, feelings of helplessness, increased cynicism, higher burnout rates, inhibition of academic advancement, feelings of isolation, depression, and higher dropout rates. [6, 15, 34, 56, 81, 92].

Assessment and Feedback

Research has found stricter standards exist for women than for men when both perform at the same level and that personality characteristics can activate different standards [33]. When attending physicians gave residents feedback regarding the trainee's performance that needed work, men received consistent feedback, whereas women residents received inconsistent feedback particularly related to autonomy and leadership [70]. There are no studies currently which have examined Milestones, a developmental framework for trainee assessment, attainment based on gender in pediatrics; however, other fields have found differences [22].

Psychological Impact of Clinical Training

During medical school, men report more worry than women [67]. However, as medical school progresses, women are noted to have both an increase in anxiety levels and an increase in reported depression all contributing to decreased psychological well-being [74, 87]. Marriage seems to serve as a social support system for men but not women during medical school [67]. Binge drinking, alcohol consumption, and marijuana and tobacco use are reported more often by men during medical school [65]. Data during pediatric training is limited but does suggest slightly higher levels of burnout among women compared to men (55% vs. 52%) [53].

Research Opportunities

Gender differences exist during both medical school and residency related to research opportunities. Although women authored a little over half of all theses in a 13-year study period, women earned only 30.9% of highest honors awards for their work [54]. Men were statistically more likely than women to work with a mentor with a history of three or more thesis honorees, undertake a fifth year of research study, secure competitive funding for their research, enroll in an MD-Master of Health Science dual degree program, and conduct bench research. Even after correcting for all these factors, women were still only half as likely to receive highest honors. In 2016, women matriculants made up only 38% of the total enrollment in Medical Scientist Training Programs, and they disproportionately apply to lower ranking research programs [2, 9]. Similar gender differences exist in research grant applications and funding among pediatric residents. Although more women than men applied (61% vs. 39%), men were more likely than women to not only obtain grant funding but also to receive more money [26]. Men tended to apply more often during their first or second year of training, propose more basic science projects, and were more likely to have an advanced research degree.

Professionalization and Professional Identity Formation

> *Are you sure you want to be a doctor? That's not what women typically do. Wouldn't you rather be a teacher or a nurse?* – Stated by multiple family members of a woman interested in going to medical school

Recent studies have hypothesized that women students are involved in a "gendered apprenticeship" where over time gender bias is internalized as the norm [12, 80]. Social norms create gendered expectations, for example, women are more likely to assume educational roles within medical schools, and these roles are often perceived as subordinate to management roles which men hold in higher numbers [29]. This gender imbalance in roles has been likened to what occurs in most households and has been labeled "institutional housekeeping" [8].

Women trainees not only walk a gender identity tightrope, but they face a double standard. Women trainees who do not conform to traditional gendered expectations risk being marginalized. Women also may be more likely to doubt their competence owing to training environments that favor more masculine behaviors [45]. When trainees live and work in an environment where images do not look like them, they also perceive that the institution does not value them [31].

Gendered experiences have a significant influence on trainees' professional identity development [12]. Women are more influenced by their ability to see themselves fitting into the specialty field (connectedness) when making career decisions [82]. Poor representation of women in some subspecialties, a paucity of role models in certain jobs, and the perception that a women's career advancement is fraught with difficulty may dissuade trainees from pursuing the same career path [12]. The proportion of first-year fellows seeking subspecialty pediatric training has increased from 50% in 2001 to almost 68% in 2018 [62]. Only two subspecialty fields, cardiology and critical care medicine, continue to have more men than women entering fellowship. There is also a positive trend of more women seeing themselves as subspecialists versus general pediatricians. In 2018, 41% of women chose to pursue pediatric fellowship, up from 34% in 2001 [62].

A lot has changed since Dr. Elizabeth Blackwell broke the mold; however, challenges still remain, and progress is ongoing. Continued dedicated efforts to remove barriers that limit women in ascending at an equivalent trajectory to men are needed and must begin at the start of the pipeline with our students. As our visibility increases, so should our voice. The contributions of women in medicine are great and their influence on the path of those women who follow is profound.

Medicine is a natural field for women. ... But if we don't have and don't utilize the capabilities of women, which are different in many ways from men, we're throwing away 50 percent, actually 51 percent, of the intellect and creativity in this country or in the world. That's wrong! – Dr. Catherine DeAngelis, M.D., M.P.H., FAAP [91]

References

1. ACGME Residents and Fellows by Sex and Specialty, 2019. AAMC. 2020, August 13. https://www.aamc.org/data-reports/interactive-data/acgme-residents-and-fellows-sex-and-specialty-2019.
2. Andrews NC. The other physician-scientist problem: where have all the young girls gone? Nat Med. 2002;8(5):439–41. https://doi.org/10.1038/nm0502-439.
3. Axelson RD, Solow CM, Ferguson KJ, Cohen MB. Assessing implicit gender bias in medical student performance evaluations. Eval Health Prof. 2010;33(3):365–85. https://doi.org/10.1177/0163278710375097.
4. Babal JC, Gower AD, Frohna JG, Moreno MA. Linguistic analysis of pediatric residency personal statements: gender differences. BMC Med Educ. 2019;19(1) https://doi.org/10.1186/s12909-019-1838-x.
5. Babaria P, Abedin S, Nunez-Smith M. The effect of gender on the clinical clerkship experiences of female medical students: results from a qualitative study. Acad Med. 2009;84(7):859–66. https://doi.org/10.1097/acm.0b013e3181a8130c.
6. Baldwin DC, Daugherty SR, Eckenfels EJ. Student perceptions of mistreatment and harassment during medical school. A survey of ten United States schools. West J Med. 1991; Published. https://www.ncbi.nlm.nih.gov/pmc/articles/PMC1002944/
7. Barzansky B, Etzel SI. Medical Schools in the United States, 2019-2020. JAMA. 2020;324(12):1220–29. https://doi.org/10.1001/jama.2020.14744.
8. Bird S, Litt J, Wang Y. Creating status of women reports: institutional housekeeping as "Women's work". NWSA J. 2004;16(1):194–206. https://doi.org/10.2979/nws.2004.16.1.194.
9. Bowen CJ, Kersbergen CJ, Tang O, Cox A, Beach MC. Medical school research ranking is associated with gender inequality in MSTP application rates. BMC Med Educ. 2018;18(1) https://doi.org/10.1186/s12909-018-1306-z.
10. Boyle P. More women than men are enrolled in medical school. AAMC. 2019, December 10. https://www.aamc.org/news-insights/more-women-men-are-enrolled-medical-school.
11. Boyle P. Nation's physician workforce evolves: more women, a bit older, and toward different specialties. AAMC. 2021, February 2. https://www.aamc.org/news-insights/nation-s-physician-workforce-evolves-more-women-bit-older-and-toward-different-specialties.
12. Brown MEL, Hunt GEG, Hughes F, Finn GM. 'Too male, too pale, too stale': a qualitative exploration of student experiences of gender bias within medical education. BMJ Open. 2020;10(8):e039092. https://doi.org/10.1136/bmjopen-2020-039092.
13. Castrillon C. Why women need to network differently than men to get ahead. Forbes. 2019, March 11. https://www.forbes.com/sites/carolinecastrillon/2019/03/10/why-women-need-to-network-differently-than-men-to-get-ahead/?sh=32205db8b0a1.
14. Colson ER., Pérez M, Blaylock L, Jeffe DB, Lawrence SJ, Wilson SA, Aagaard EM. Washington University School of Medicine in St. Louis Case Study: a process for understanding and addressing bias in clerkship grading. Acad Med. 2020;95(12S Addressing Harmful Bias and Eliminating Discrimination in Health Professions Learning Environments), S131–5. https://doi.org/10.1097/ACM.0000000000003702.
15. Cook AF, Arora VM, Rasinski KA, Curlin FA, Yoon JD. The prevalence of medical student mistreatment and its association with burnout. Acad Med. 2014;89(5):749–54. https://doi.org/10.1097/acm.0000000000000204.

16. Cook DJ, Liutkus JF, Risdon CL, Griffith LE, Guyatt GH, Walter SD. Residents' experiences of abuse, discrimination and sexual harassment during residency training. McMaster University Residency Training Programs. CMAJ. 1996:1657–65. https://pubmed.ncbi.nlm.nih.gov/8646653/
17. Cortina LM, Jagsi R. What can medicine learn from social science studies of sexual harassment? Ann Intern Med. 2018;169(10):716. https://doi.org/10.7326/m18-2047.
18. Craig LB, Smith C, Crow SM, Driver W, Wallace M, Thompson BM. Obstetrics and gynecology clerkship for males and females: similar curriculum, different outcomes? Med Educ Online. 2013;18:21506. https://doi.org/10.3402/meo.v18i0.21506.
19. Crebbin W, Campbell G, Hillis DA, Watters DA. Prevalence of bullying, discrimination and sexual harassment in surgery in Australasia. ANZ J Surg. 2015;85(12):905–9. https://doi.org/10.1111/ans.13363.
20. Crowe S, Clarke N, Brugha R. 'You do not cross them': hierarchy and emotion in doctors' narratives of power relations in specialist training. Soc Sci Med. 2017;186:70–7. https://doi.org/10.1016/j.socscimed.2017.05.048.
21. Cusimano MC, Baxter NN, Sutradhar R, McArthur E, Ray JG, Garg AX, Vigod S, Simpson AN. Delay of pregnancy among physicians vs nonphysicians. JAMA Intern Med. Published. 2021; https://doi.org/10.1001/jamainternmed.2021.1635.
22. Dayal A, O'Connor DM, Qadri U, Arora VM. Comparison of male vs female resident milestone evaluations by faculty during emergency medicine residency training. JAMA Intern Med. 2017;177(5):651. https://doi.org/10.1001/jamainternmed.2016.9616.
23. Demzik A, Filippou P, Chew C, Deal A, Mercer E, Mahajan S, Wallen EM, Tan HJ, Smith AB. Gender-based differences in urology residency applicant personal statements. Urology. 2021;150:2–8. https://doi.org/10.1016/j.urology.2020.08.066.
24. Eagly AH, Johannesen-Schmidt MC, van Engen ML. Transformational, transactional, and laissez-faire leadership styles: a meta-analysis comparing women and men. Psychol Bull. 2003;129(4):569–91. https://doi.org/10.1037/0033-2909.129.4.569.
25. Eagly AH, Karau SJ. Role congruity theory of prejudice toward female leaders. Psychol Rev. 2002;109(3):573–98. https://doi.org/10.1037/0033-295x.109.3.573.
26. Gordon MB, Osganian SK, Emans SJ, Lovejoy FH Jr. Gender differences in research grant applications for pediatric residents. Pediatrics. 2009;124(2):e355–61. https://doi.org/10.1542/peds.2008-3626.
27. Gorth DJ, Magee RG, Rosenberg SE, Mingioni N. Gender disparity in evaluation of internal medicine clerkship performance. JAMA Netw Open. 2021;4(7):e2115661. https://doi.org/10.1001/jamanetworkopen.2021.15661.
28. Fatherly. This is what kids in 2015 want to be when they grow up. Fatherly. 2020, August 14. https://www.fatherly.com/news/what-kids-want-to-be-when-they-grow-up/.
29. Farid H. Hidden costs of motherhood in medicine. Obstet Gynecol. 2019;134(6):1339–41. https://doi.org/10.1097/aog.0000000000003575.
30. Filippou P, Mahajan S, Deal A, Wallen EM, Tan HJ, Pruthi RS, Smith AB. The presence of gender bias in letters of recommendations written for urology residency applicants. Urology. 2019;134:56–61. https://doi.org/10.1016/j.urology.2019.05.065.
31. Fitzsousa E, Anderson N, Reisman A. "This institution was never meant for me": the impact of institutional historical portraiture on medical students. J Gen Intern Med. 2019;34(12):2738–9. https://doi.org/10.1007/s11606-019-05138-9.
32. Fnais N, Soobiah C, Chen MH, Lillie E, Perrier L, Tashkhandi M, Straus SE, Mamdani M, Al-Omran M, Tricco AC. Harassment and discrimination in medical training. Acad Med. 2014;89(5):817–27. https://doi.org/10.1097/acm.0000000000000200.
33. Foschi M. Double standards for competence: theory and research. Annu Rev Sociol. 2000;26(1):21–42. https://doi.org/10.1146/annurev.soc.26.1.21.
34. Frank E, Brogan D, Schiffman M. Prevalence and correlates of harassment among US women physicians. Arch Intern Med. 1998;158(4):352. https://doi.org/10.1001/archinte.158.4.352.

35. Fried JM, Vermillion M, Parker NH, Uijtdehaage S. Eradicating medical student mistreatment. Acad Med. 2012;87(9):1191–8. https://doi.org/10.1097/acm.0b013e3182625408.
36. Grimm LJ, Redmond RA, Campbell JC, Rosette AS. Gender and racial bias in radiology residency letters of recommendation. J Am Coll Radiol. 2020;17(1):64–71. https://doi.org/10.1016/j.jacr.2019.08.008.
37. Grover A, Appelbaum N, Santen SA, Lee N, Hemphill RR, Goldberg S. Physician mistreatment in the clinical learning environment. Am J Surg. 2020;220(2):276–81. https://doi.org/10.1016/j.amjsurg.2019.11.038.
38. Haggins AN. To be seen, heard, and valued: strategies to promote a sense of belonging for women and underrepresented in medicine physicians. Acad Med. 2020;95(10):1507–10. https://doi.org/10.1097/acm.0000000000003553.
39. Halim UA, Riding DM. Systematic review of the prevalence, impact and mitigating strategies for bullying, undermining behaviour and harassment in the surgical workplace. Br J Surg. 2018;105(11):1390–7. https://doi.org/10.1002/bjs.10926.
40. Hammoud MM, Appelbaum NP, Wallach PM, Burrows HL, Kochhar K, Hemphill RR, Daniel M, Clery MJ, Santen SA. Incidence of resident mistreatment in the learning environment across three institutions. Med Teach. 2021;43(3):334–40. https://doi.org/10.1080/0142159x.2020.1845306.
41. Having a Baby After Age 35: How Aging Affects Fertility and Pregnancy. ACOG. 2020. https://www.acog.org/womens-health/faqs/having-a-baby-after-age-35-how-aging-affects-fertility-and-pregnancy.
42. Heilman ME. Description and prescription: how gender stereotypes prevent women's ascent up the organizational ladder. J Soc Issues. 2001;57(4):657–74. https://doi.org/10.1111/0022-4537.00234.
43. Heilman ME, Okimoto TG. Why are women penalized for success at male tasks?: the implied communality deficit. J Appl Psychol. 2007;92(1):81–92. https://doi.org/10.1037/0021-9010.92.1.81.
44. Heilman ME, Wallen AS, Fuchs D, Tamkins MM. Penalties for success: reactions to women who succeed at male gender-typed tasks. J Appl Psychol. 2004;89(3):416–27. https://doi.org/10.1037/0021-9010.89.3.416.
45. Hingle S, Barrett E. Gender Differences in Resident Assessment. JAMA Netw Open. 2020;3(7):e2010985. https://doi.org/10.1001/jamanetworkopen.2020.10985.
46. Hoff T. The challenges of being a female doctor. Medical Economics. 2020, November 12. https://www.medicaleconomics.com/view/challenges-being-female-doctor.
47. Hoff T, Scott S. The gendered realities and talent management imperatives of women physicians. Health Care Manag Rev. 2016;41(3):189–99. https://doi.org/10.1097/hmr.0000000000000069.
48. Hoffman A, Grant W, McCormick M, Jezewski E, Matemavi P, Langnas A. Gendered differences in letters of recommendation for transplant surgery fellowship applicants. J Surg Educ. 2019;76(2):427–32. https://doi.org/10.1016/j.jsurg.2018.08.021.
49. Horowitz JM, Igielnik R. A century after women gained the right to vote, majority of Americans see work to do on gender equality. Pew Research Center's Social & Demographic Trends Project. 2020, July 7. https://www.pewresearch.org/social-trends/2020/07/07/a-century-after-women-gained-the-right-to-vote-majority-of-americans-see-work-to-do-on-gender-equality/.
50. Hu YY, Ellis RJ, Hewitt DB, Yang AD, Cheung EO, Moskowitz JT, Potts JR, Buyske J, Hoyt DB, Nasca TJ, Bilimoria KY. Discrimination, abuse, harassment, and burnout in surgical residency training. N Engl J Med. 2019;381(18):1741–52. https://doi.org/10.1056/nejmsa1903759.
51. Jagsi R. Sexual harassment in medicine — #MeToo. N Engl J Med. 2018;378(3):209–11. https://doi.org/10.1056/nejmp1715962.
52. Kemper KJ, Schwartz A. Bullying, discrimination, sexual harassment, and physical violence: common and associated with burnout in pediatric residents. Acad Pediatr. 2020;20(7):991–7. https://doi.org/10.1016/j.acap.2020.02.023.

53. Kemper KJ, Schwartz A, Wilson PM, Mahan JD, Schubert CJ, Staples BB, McClafferty H, Serwint JR, Batra M, Pediatric Resident Burnout-Resilience Study Consortium. Burnout in Pediatric residents: three years of National Survey Data. Pediatrics. 2020;145(1):e20191030. https://doi.org/10.1542/peds.2019-1030.
54. King JT, Angoff NR, Forrest JN, Justice AC. Gender disparities in medical student research awards. Acad Med. 2018;93(6):911–9. https://doi.org/10.1097/acm.0000000000002052.
55. Kolehmainen C, Brennan M, Filut A, Isaac C, Carnes M. Afraid of being "witchy with a 'B'". Acad Med. 2014;89(9):1276–81. https://doi.org/10.1097/acm.0000000000000372.
56. Komaromy M, Bindman AB, Haber RJ, Sande MA. Sexual harassment in medical training. N Engl J Med. 1993;329(9):661–3. https://doi.org/10.1056/nejm199308263290914.
57. Larsson C, Hensing G, Allebeck P. Sexual and gender-related harassment in medical education and research training: results from a Swedish survey. Med Educ. 2003;37(1):39–50. https://doi.org/10.1046/j.1365-2923.2003.01404.x.
58. Li SF, Grant K, Bhoj T, Lent G, Garrick JF, Greenwald P, Haber M, Singh M, Prodany K, Sanchez L, Dickman E, Spencer J, Perera T, Cowan E. Resident experience of abuse and harassment in emergency medicine: ten years later. J Emerg Med. 2010;38(2):248–52. https://doi.org/10.1016/j.jemermed.2008.05.005.
59. Li S, Fant AL, McCarthy DM, Miller D, Craig J, Kontrick A. Gender differences in language of standardized letter of evaluation narratives for emergency medicine residency applicants. AEM Educat Training. 2017;1(4):334–9. https://doi.org/10.1002/aet2.10057.
60. Lin F, Oh SK, Gordon LK, Pineles SL, Rosenberg JB, Tsui I. Gender-based differences in letters of recommendation written for ophthalmology residency applicants. BMC Med Educ. 2019;19(1) https://doi.org/10.1186/s12909-019-1910-6.
61. Llewellyn A, Karageorge A, Nash L, Li W, Neuen D. Bullying and sexual harassment of junior doctors in New South Wales, Australia: rate and reporting outcomes. Aust Health Rev. 2019;43(3):328. https://doi.org/10.1071/ah17224.
62. Macy ML, Leslie LK, Turner A, Freed GL. Growth and changes in the pediatric medical subspecialty workforce pipeline. Pediatr Res. 2021;89(5):1297–303. https://doi.org/10.1038/s41390-020-01311-7.
63. Main Residency Match Data and Reports. The Match, National Resident Matching Program. 2021, September 28. https://www.nrmp.org/main-residency-match-data/.
64. Mann A, Denis V, Schleicher A, Ekhtiari H, Forsyth T, Liu E, OECD Publishing. Teenagers' career aspirations and the future of work. OECD.Org. 2020. https://www.oecd.org/education/dream-jobs-teenagers-career-aspirations-and-the-future-of-work.htm.
65. Merlo LJ, Curran JS, Watson R. Gender differences in substance use and psychiatric distress among medical students: a comprehensive statewide evaluation. Subst Abus. 2017;38(4):401–6. https://doi.org/10.1080/08897077.2017.1355871.
66. Microys G. Women as doctors, wives, and mothers. Can Fam Physician. 1986:339–42. https://www.ncbi.nlm.nih.gov/pmc/articles/PMC2328102/
67. Miller GD, Kemmelmeier M, Dupey P. Gender differences in worry during medical school. Med Educ. 2013;47(9):932–41. https://doi.org/10.1111/medu.12236.
68. Moorkamp M. Women paediatricians: what made them choose their career? J Health Organ Manag. 2005;19(6):478–93. https://doi.org/10.1108/14777260510629652.
69. Moss-Racusin CA, Rudman LA. Disruptions in women's self-promotion: the backlash avoidance model. Psychol Women Q. 2010;34(2):186–202. https://doi.org/10.1111/j.1471-6402.2010.01561.x.
70. Mueller AS, Jenkins TM, Osborne M, Dayal A, O'Connor DM, Arora VM. Gender differences in attending physicians' feedback to residents: a qualitative analysis. J Grad Med Educ. 2017;9(5):577–85. https://doi.org/10.4300/jgme-d-17-00126.1.
71. Nora LM, McLaughlin MA, Fosson SE, Stratton TD, Murphy-Spencer A, Fincher RME, German DC, Seiden D, Witzke DB. Gender discrimination and sexual harassment in medical education. Acad Med. 2002;77(12, Part 1):1226–34. https://doi.org/10.1097/00001888-200212000-00018

72. Osman NY, Schonhardt-Bailey C, Walling JL, Katz JT, Alexander EK. Textual analysis of internal medicine residency personal statements: themes and gender differences. Med Educ. 2015;49(1):93–102. https://doi.org/10.1111/medu.12487.
73. Ostapenko L, Schonhardt-Bailey C, Sublette JW, Smink DS, Osman NY. Textual analysis of general surgery residency personal statements: topics and gender differences. J Surg Educ. 2018;75(3):573–81. https://doi.org/10.1016/j.jsurg.2017.09.021.
74. Rosal MC, Ockene IS, Ockene JK, Barrett SV, Ma Y, Hebert JR. A longitudinal study of students' depression at one medical school. Acad Med. 1997;72(6):542–6. https://doi.org/10.1097/00001888-199706000-00022.
75. Ross DA, Boatright D, Nunez-Smith M, Jordan A, Chekroud A, Moore EZ. Differences in words used to describe racial and gender groups in medical student performance evaluations. PLoS One. 2017;12(8):e0181659. https://doi.org/10.1371/journal.pone.0181659.
76. Rosser VJ. Faculty and staff members' perceptions of effective leadership: are there differences between women and men leaders? Equity Excell Educ. 2003;36(1):71–81. https://doi.org/10.1080/10665680303501.
77. Rubright JD, Jodoin M, Barone MA. Examining demographics, prior academic performance, and United States medical licensing examination scores. Acad Med. 2019;94(3):364–70. https://doi.org/10.1097/acm.0000000000002366.
78. Rudman LA, Glick P. Prescriptive gender stereotypes and backlash toward agentic women. J Soc Issues. 2001;57(4):743–62. https://doi.org/10.1111/0022-4537.00239.
79. Rudman LA, Kilianski SE. Implicit and explicit attitudes toward female authority. Personal Soc Psychol Bull. 2000;26(11):1315–28. https://doi.org/10.1177/0146167200263001.
80. Samuriwo R, Patel Y, Webb K, Bullock A. 'Man up': medical students' perceptions of gender and learning in clinical practice: a qualitative study. Med Educ. 2020;54(2):150–61. https://doi.org/10.1111/medu.13959.
81. Sheehan KH. A pilot study of medical student "abuse". Student perceptions of mistreatment and misconduct in medical school. J Am Med Assoc. 1990;263(4):533–7. https://doi.org/10.1001/jama.263.4.533.
82. Smith V, Bethune C, Hurley KF. Examining medical student specialty choice through a gender lens: an Orientational qualitative study. Teach Learn Med. 2018;30(1):33–44. https://doi.org/10.1080/10401334.2017.1306447.
83. Spector ND, Cull W, Daniels SR, Gilhooly J, Hall J, Horn I, Marshall SG, Schumacher DJ, Sectish TC, Stanton BF. Gender and generational influences on the pediatric workforce and practice. Pediatrics. 2014;133(6):1112–21. https://doi.org/10.1542/peds.2013-3016.
84. Trix F, Psenka C. Exploring the color of glass: letters of recommendation for female and male medical faculty. Discourse Soc. 2003;14(2):191–220. https://doi.org/10.1177/0957926503014002277.
85. Tsugawa Y, Jena AB, Figueroa JF, Orav EJ, Blumenthal DM, Jha AK. Comparison of hospital mortality and readmission rates for Medicare patients treated by male vs female physicians. JAMA Intern Med. 2017;177(2):206. https://doi.org/10.1001/jamainternmed.2016.7875.
86. Turrentine FE, Dreisbach CN, St Ivany AR, Hanks JB, Schroen AT. Influence of gender on surgical residency applicants' recommendation letters. J Am Coll Surg. 2019;228(4):356–365.e3. https://doi.org/10.1016/j.jamcollsurg.2018.12.020.
87. Vitaliano PP, Maiuro RD, Russo J, Mitchell ES. Medical student distress: a longitudinal study. J Nerv Ment Dis. 1989;177(2):70–6. https://doi.org/10.1097/00005053-198902000-00002.
88. Wayne NL, Vermillion M, Uijtdehaage S. Gender differences in leadership amongst first-year medical students in the small-group setting. Acad Med. 2010;85(8):1276–81. https://doi.org/10.1097/acm.0b013e3181e5f2ce.
89. Wijesekera TP, Kim M, Moore EZ, Sorenson O, Ross DA. All other things being equal. Acad Med. 2019;94(4):562–9. https://doi.org/10.1097/acm.0000000000002463.
90. Women Chairs of the Association of Medical School Pediatric Department Chairs. Women in pediatrics: recommendations for the future. American Academy of Pediatrics. 2007, May 1. https://pediatrics.aappublications.org/content/119/5/1000?download=true.

91. Wyckoff AS. In their words: quotes from the AAP oral histories of 10 female pediatricians. American Academy of Pediatrics. 2019, May 9. https://www.aappublications.org/news/2019/05/09/dyk050919.
92. Yaghmour A, Alesa A, Anbarserry E, Abdullah Binmerdah M, Alharbi A, Housawi A, Almehdar M, Lytra H, Alsaywid B, Lytras DM. Challenges and obstacles faced by trainee female physicians: an integrative research on gender discrimination, stress, depression and harassment. Healthcare. 2021;9(2):160. https://doi.org/10.3390/healthcare90.

Chapter 3
Women Practicing in Pediatrics

Eleanor Sharp, Catherine Forster, Samir Shah, and Kayce Morton

Workforce Trends

The number of women in medicine has increased over the past several decades. The 2003–2004 academic year was the first time that more women than men applied to medical school, and in 2007–2008, 49% of medical school graduates were women [4]. In the 2018–2019 academic year, women comprised 50.9% of all applicants to medical school, 51.6% of medical school matriculants, and 47.9% of graduates [4]. Women make up 45.6% of all medical residents in the United States yet comprised only 36% of full-time medical school faculty in 2009 and 41% of all medical school faculty in 2018 [4]. Further, there is a decreasing proportion of women at each increase in faculty rank: in 2018, 58% of instructors, 46% of assistant professors, 37% of associate professors, and 25% of full professors were women [4]. Physicians

E. Sharp · C. Forster (✉)
UPMC Children's Hospital of Pittsburgh, University of Pittsburgh, Pittsburgh, PA, USA
e-mail: eleanor.sharp@chp.edu; forstercs@upmc.edu

S. Shah
Division of Hospital Medicine, Cincinnati Children's Hospital Medical Center, Cincinnati, OH, USA

Department of Pediatrics, University of Cincinnati College of Medicine, Cincinnati, OH, USA
e-mail: Samir.shah@cchmc.org

K. Morton
Jordan Valley Community Health Center, Cox Health, Springfield, MO, USA
e-mail: Kayce.morton@coxhealth.com

N. D. Spector et al. (eds.), *Women in Pediatrics*,
https://doi.org/10.1007/978-3-030-98222-5_3

who are women are also more likely to remain in the assistant professor role compared with their counterparts who are men [68] (Fig. 3.1). Further, women physicians with children receive less institutional support and have decreased academic

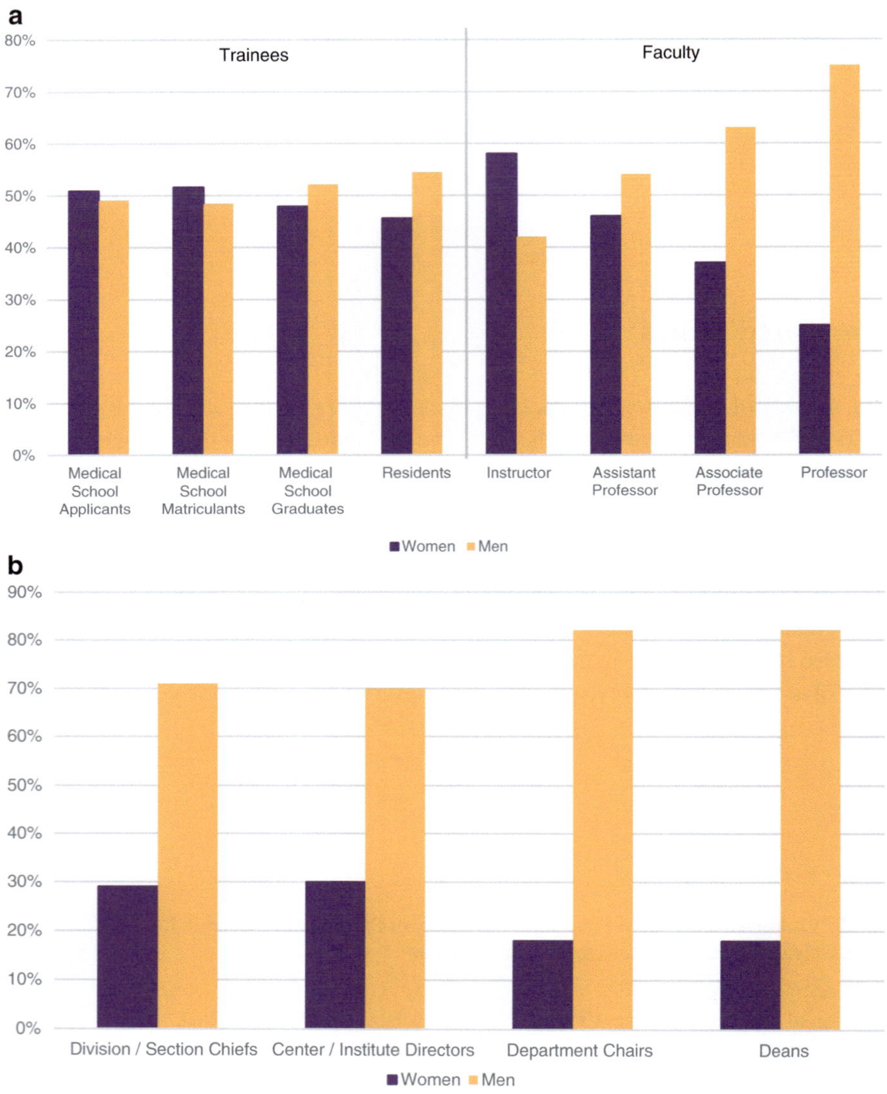

Fig. 3.1 (**a**) Proportion of women and men at each stage of medical training (left side of figure), and on faculty at medical schools in the United States in the 2018–2019 academic year. While the proportion of women who are medical school applicants and matriculants are higher than men, there are more men who graduate medical school and who are residents. Among faculty at medical schools in the United States, the only rank in which there are more women than men is instructor. (Data from the State of Women in Academic Medicine: 2018–2019, published by the Association of American Medical Colleges, 2019). (**b**) Proportion of women who hold various leadership positions within American medical schools. There are more men than women in each of the included positions. (Data from the State of Women in Academic Medicine: 2018–2019, published by the Association of American Medical Colleges, 2019)

productivity compared with colleagues with children who are men [20]. The COVID-19 pandemic has only exacerbated these existing gender gaps, with recent work showing that women faculty with children were more likely than those without children to consider leaving academic medicine [57].

The trend of gender inequity in academic medicine continues into leadership, as women are also underrepresented in both divisional and departmental leadership within medical schools. Only 29% of division chiefs and 18% of department chairs in 2018 were women [4]. As expected, the same trend continues with medical school deans. In 2017, only 16.9% of deans were women [74] (Fig. 3.1b). Further, women who were deans were more likely to be in positions focused on education or mentorship or in positions related to maintaining the public image of the institution, whereas deans who are men were more likely to be focused on strategy, policy, finance, and government relations [72].

Women in Academic Pediatrics

According to the 2020 Physician Specialty Data Report from the Association of American Medical Colleges, women account for 36.4% of all practicing physicians in the United States, but 64.3% of all pediatricians [9]. Despite the preponderance of women in pediatrics, only 27.5% of pediatric department chairs were women in 2018, suggesting that the lack of representation of women in the higher echelons of academic medicine persists regardless of the gender distribution of the field at large. Even outside of academic leadership, there are persistent decreases in the proportion of women from training to practice, as 72.3% of pediatric residents in 2017 were women, compared with 63.3% of pediatricians out of training and 57.4% of those in academic pediatrics. According to the American Academy of Medical Colleges, women accounted for 70% of instructors, 60% of assistant professors, 48% of associate professors, and 32% of full professors in the pediatric departments in 2015 [2]. However, there is variability among different subspecialities within pediatrics. For example, in neonatology, women comprise 46% of assistant professors, 27% of associate professors, and 15% of full professors [45], whereas in pediatric ophthalmology, 64.4% of assistant professors, 21.7% of associate professors, and 13.9% of full professors are women [18]. Part of the difficulty in obtaining accurate data on rank is the wide array of pediatric subspecialities and the lack of a central repository for such data. The inability to accurately track trends in gender across institutions within the broader field of pediatrics is a major limiting factor to advancing gender equity.

There are several theories as to the reasons for the differences in gender distribution in academic medicine: (1) women are less interested in research than men or become less interested in research as they advance in their careers; (2) women are more interested in teaching than research; (3) there is a lack of role models and mentors for women; (4) financial considerations lead women to leave academia; (5) concerns about work-life balance lead women to leave academia; and (6) gender discrimination and unconscious bias force women to leave academia [28] (Fig. 3.2).

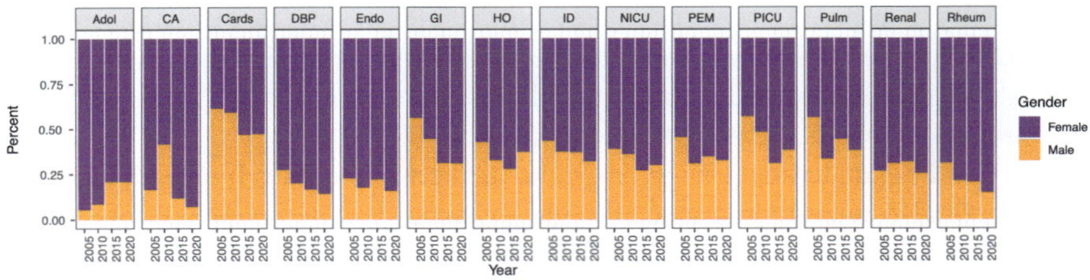

Fig. 3.2 Proportion of first-year fellows who are men and women in pediatric fellowships over a 15-year period (2005 to 2020). Adol, adolescent medicine; CA, child abuse pediatrics; Cards, cardiology; DBP, development behavioral pediatrics; Endo, endocrinology; GI, gastroenterology; HO, hematology oncology; ID, infectious diseases; NICU, neonatology and newborn medicine; PEM, pediatric emergency medicine; PICU, critical care medicine; Pulm, pulmonology; Renal, nephrology; Rheum, rheumatology. (Data from the American Board of Pediatrics, Research Department (2021). Data sent on April 30, 2021, related to https://www.abp.org/content/data-and-workforce. Chapel Hill, NC: The American Board of Pediatrics)

However, evidence supporting these theories are conflicting. Of these six categories, only three are universally supported in the literature: women are more interested in teaching than research; lack of role models/mentors for women; and the existence of gender bias and unconscious discrimination [28]. One institutional study of a large department of pediatrics found that although there was not a gender-based disparity in the proportion of men and women at either the assistant or associate professor level, professors who were men had been at their current rank for 6 years more than women and were promoted from assistant to associate professor faster than their women counterparts [70]. Others have found similar trends in lack of promotion, and have hypothesized that women spend more time than men in tasks that are not directly related to promotion. Indeed, women spend more time per week engaged in teaching activities, whereas men spend more time directly engaged in research or advising faculty members [62]. This same institution performed a local gender equity study, and identified gender-based disparities in the domains of tenure, leadership roles, faculty retention, and salary. For tenure, they noted that they hired fewer women faculty with tenure and granted fewer women tenure with promotion. They also noted a higher rate of women than men who either resigned or relocated [70].

There are conflicting data on women in research in medicine with evidence suggesting that although the same proportion of women and men are interested in research at the beginning of training, this may change over time [17]. One study found that women were less likely than men to graduate from an MD/PhD program [7]. However, the reasons behind this attrition were not clear. For women in academic pediatrics engaged in research, gender disparities persist despite the increased number of women in the field. Analysis of research publications found that 58% of first authors and 38% of senior authors of original research articles in three major pediatric journals were women [31]. Although these rates are improved from 2001 (when 40% of first authors and 29% of senior authors were women), disparities remain [31]. Similarly, a study of publications in the four journals with the highest impact factors in general pediatrics found that women were underrepresented as first authors and that this disparity in first authorship was more prominent in scholarly as opposed to narrative article types [73]. In summary, despite comprising most of the workforce, women pediatricians are less likely than their colleagues who are men to receive research funding, publish both original research and perspective-type articles, and receive invited commentaries and professorships [31, 73].

Women in General Pediatrics

According to the American Board of Pediatrics, most pediatricians practice general outpatient pediatrics (54.9%), the majority of whom are women (59.2% women vs 48.4% men) and do not have an academic appointment (60% of women who practice general pediatrics do not have an academic appointment) [65]. Of the remaining 40% of women in general pediatrics, 25% are adjunct faculty, and 14% are academic faculty (8% full time, 6% part time). Few women (0.7%) in general pediatrics work primarily in industry [65]. There are several notable gender-based differences among general pediatricians. First, women in general pediatrics have 12-fold greater odds of working part time compared with men. Further, women in general pediatrics are less likely to feel that the distribution of their professional time is what they want compared to men. Finally, women were more likely than men to anticipate retiring before the age of 65 years [35].

Women in Subspecialties

The proportion of pediatric residents who are women has been largely unchanged since 2007, with women comprising between 70 and 72% of all pediatric residents [64]. Comparatively, in the past two decades, there has been an increase in the proportion of first-year pediatric fellows who are women. Women represented 50% of first-year fellows in 2001 and 68% in 2018 [56]. This corresponds to 41% of all residents who are women who enter fellowship in 2018, an increase from 34% in 2009. Comparatively, 50% and 49% of residents who are men entered fellowship in 2009 and 2018, respectively [56]. Only two pediatric subspecialities, cardiology and critical care, had more men than women enter fellowship within the study period [56] (Fig. 3.3).

Workforce trends for pediatric subspecialists are similar to those in general pediatrics. Among pediatric subspecialists, 44% of women had full-time academic appointments, compared with 49% of men [36]. Women in pediatric subspecialities were also less likely to have jobs that met their ideal professional duties [36] and were six times more likely to work part time compared with men. Finally, women in subspecialties were more likely to anticipate retiring before the age of 65 compared with men [36].

Practice Setting

Only a small proportion of women in outpatient pediatrics are full owners of their practice (28%), while 34% are part owner and 38% do not own their practice [60]. Further, women are more likely than men to be employees as opposed to practice owners [5]. The decision whether to pursue a career in an academic setting or private practice is complex and has been the subject of multiple studies. Individuals with higher student loan burden may elect to pursue a private practice position with higher compensation. Perceived barriers to working in private practice include concern about work-life balance, lack of training in coding and billing, lack of training in practice management, and desire to avoid malpractice insurance premiums [66]. However, clinicians in private practices have higher career satisfaction than those in hospital- or corporate-owned practices [37]. Despite the potential financial benefits of private practice, there is an increasing trend in physicians moving away from private practice and into hospital- or corporate-owned practices where physicians are employees rather than owners.

Proposed Drivers of Gender Disparity in Pediatrics

The field of pediatrics has a high proportion of women. However, even in a field in which women outnumber men, women are underrepresented in certain pediatric subspecialties. Are women motivated to pursue certain fields but driven away due to obstacles? What are these obstacles, and what can be done to overcome them for

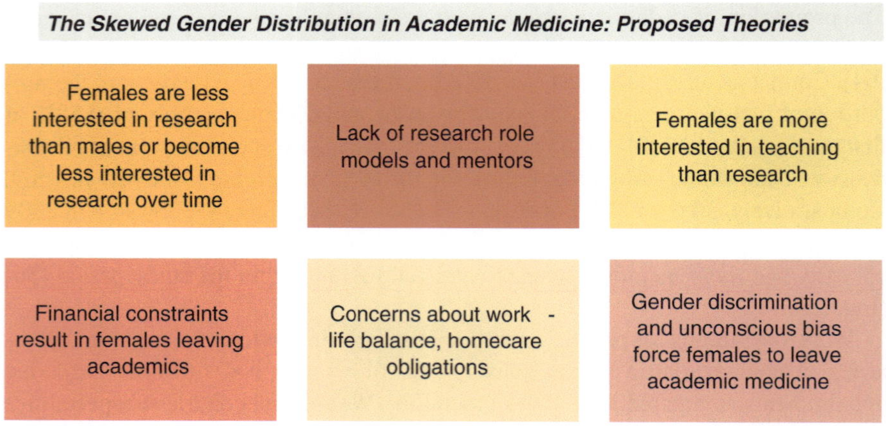

Fig. 3.3 Various theories have been proposed to explain the skewed gender distribution in academic medicine

future generations? Potential drivers may include gender bias and discrimination training during medical school and residency, availability of women faculty mentors and faculty allies who are men, and challenges achieving work-life integration that are unique to women.

Childbearing and Rearing

Medical training coincides with peak fertility and childbearing years, as the average age of the matriculating medical student is 24 years [3]. Age and stage of life at the time of entering training may affect career choice. Medical students with children have less schedule flexibility, incur high childcare expenses, and have increased homecare responsibilities [27]. Additionally, women trainees interested in starting or growing their family through pregnancy or adoption may have different priorities than their counterparts who are men. Physicians are more likely to delay childbirth than nonphysicians, with subspecialty physicians tending to further delay childbirth until completion of training [26]. Unfortunately, many women physicians suffer consequences of delaying childbirth for their career: the infertility rate among the American physicians who are women is twice that of the general population [77].

Further complicating family planning for women pediatricians are the complexities of parental leave, breastfeeding, and childcare during training. Maternity leave standards vary across specialties, institutions, and training programs [47]; trainees faced with the threat of having to extend training due to pregnancy may reconsider further sub-specialization. Without consistent, transparent, universal policies, women trainees are left to speculate whether maternity leave will jeopardize their board eligibility and employment opportunities. This uncertainty can create conflict between family planning and career planning.

Personal Factors

Many women pediatricians enter the workforce with young children and are more likely than physicians who are men to have partners who work full time [39]. Thus, personal factors, such as geographic proximity to family, schedule predictability, loan repayment obligations, and a partner's employment status, may influence career decisions for women in pediatrics [16, 38]. Among 238 pediatric residents interviewed between 1991 and 2002, lifestyle was significantly more important to women residents' career choice, and women were significantly more likely to choose generalist careers when compared with their counterparts who were men [44]. Additional lifestyle factors include salary, which may be more important for single-income families, single mothers, or women with high student loan burdens.

Gender Bias and Segregation

Gender stereotypes are a significant driver of disparities. Women are traditionally expected to adhere to social norms of being compassionate caregivers. When applied to medicine, gender stereotypes disadvantage women physicians. While women physicians are expected to be caring, approachable, and collaborative, physicians who are men are assertive, powerful, and technically skilled. Women physicians that fit the gender stereotype of being gentle and caring are generally more "liked," but less likely to be considered for leadership positions. Contrarily, women that exhibit traditionally "masculine" traits such as assertiveness and ambition are more likely to be regarded as "aggressive," "abrupt," or "emotional." This "likability paradox" results in women being less likely to be considered for leadership positions or promotion compared to colleagues who are men [23].

Implicit gender bias, or so-called second-generation gender bias, starts in medical school; women medical students are more likely to receive evaluations based on personal attributes rather than clinical or procedural competency and are more likely to struggle to identify mentors or receive advice to consider alternative careers to maintain work-life balance [41, 46, 49, 50, 66, 69] . Additionally, women medical students may experience "stereotype threat" when the fear or anxiety of being judged or confirming a negative stereotype paradoxically undermines performance [75].

Gender segregation and bias persist after medical school to create inequity at all career stages (Fig. 3.4). Young women faculty are less likely to negotiate for salary, research funding, and protected time during the job search process [19, 32]. Subsequently, once employed as junior faculty, women physicians are more likely to be tasked with uncompensated, non-promotable work such as serving on committees, organizing events, and teaching trainees while simultaneously bearing a disproportionate amount of homecare responsibilities.

Gender discrimination, sexual harassment, salary inequities, under-recognition, and challenges with work-life integration can lead to women pediatricians feeling disconnected and disillusioned. Women physicians are more likely to report burnout than physicians who are men [58]. A significant driver is the unequal distribution of traditional domestic tasks between men and women. Women pediatricians are more likely than pediatricians who are men to report being primarily responsible for household responsibilities [76]. Indeed, women spend an additional 8.5 hours per week on childcare, eldercare, and other homecare responsibilities [48]. Thus, women pediatricians often require more schedule flexibility than their counterparts who are men. In fact, women that feel less in control of their work environment and over their schedule report more career dissatisfaction and burnout [33]. On average, women physicians work 50.28 hours per week, while physicians who are men work an average of 54.12 hours per week [60]. Additionally, women physicians are more likely to work part time, with as many as 20% of pediatric residents seeking part-time employment after residency graduation [25]. In 2018, 10% of all physicians were working part time (30 hours or less) [1]. Meanwhile, 22.6% of women physicians reported that they were not working full time within 6 years of training compared with only 3.6% of physicians who were men [34].

Mentoring relationships can have substantial impacts on specialty choice, career development, and job satisfaction, and can help mitigate burnout among physicians [67]. Gender-based power dynamics and stereotypes influence the way students experience mentorship which can make mentoring relationships less satisfying and more challenging for women. Additionally, because of the leaky pipeline of women in academic medicine and the gender segregation of multiple pediatric subspecialties, it can be challenging for mentees to identify women mentors. Lack of mentorship has been described as a barrier to career development and job satisfaction for women in medicine [12, 52, 53, 59]. Fortunately, relational mentoring, or mentoring relationships that promote mutual career development, has been found to be more important than gender concordance for many mentor-mentee relationships [30, 53], underscoring the importance of the allyship of men. Additional facilitators of effective mentoring include mentor availability and experience, responsiveness, and mutual trust [53, 59]. Formal mentoring programs can reduce barriers to mentorship and promote career advancement for physicians who are women.

Salary

Women physicians earn less than men in every specialty and at every academic rank in medicine [42], and the pay gap in medicine is one of the largest in the US labor market [43]. Salary expectations and negotiations during initial hiring can

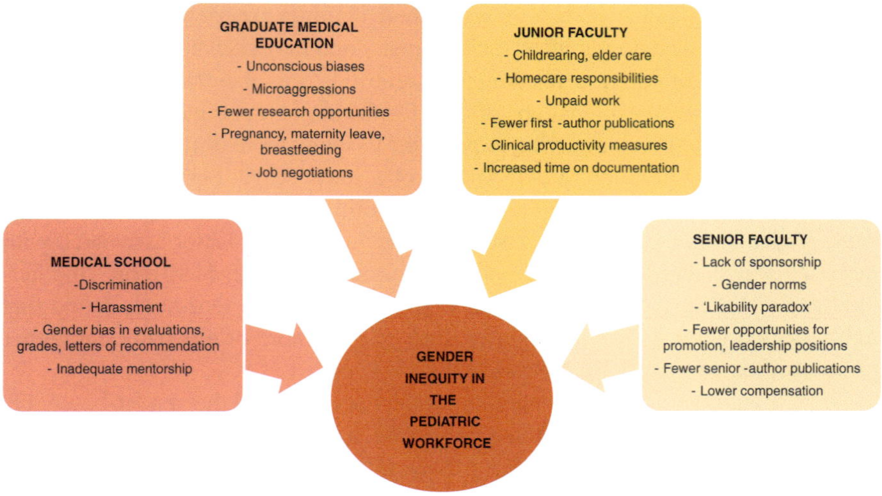

Fig. 3.4 Different factors contribute to gender inequities throughout all stages of a pediatrician's career, from medical school to senior professorship

determine both current salary and future earnings, and are the initial points at which the pay gap between women and men, which can have considerable long-term financial impact, begins [61]. Lifetime earning potential is already lower for pediatrician generalists and pediatric subspecialists compared to adult physicians, even when adjusting for the shorter training durations typical of adult medicine [22]. While differences in duration of training (and duration of loan repayment deferrals) contributes to these discrepancies, differences in salaries are far more significant [21, 22]. Medical students, especially those with children, debt, or other financial obligations, may be less likely to pursue specialties that require longer duration of training without the promise of increased earning potential. Over time, this may result in fewer trainees pursuing pediatrics.

Of further concern is recent data suggesting that the amount of compensation is inversely related to the proportion of women in a specialty [13, 66], with the field of pediatrics serving as a prime example. Research into the effect of gender distribution on salary found that there was an association between the proportion of women in a specific field and salary, with specialties with the highest proportion of women earning the lowest salaries [13]. This association is borne out in pediatrics, a field dominated by women. Women in both general pediatrics and subspecialties have a lower salary than men in the same fields [40], with an unadjusted annual difference of $51,319 between the salaries of men and women. After adjusting for a comprehensive set of job-related factors and specific work-family characteristics, this difference dropped to just under $8000 per year [40]. However, this disparity in salary adds up over the course of a physician's career, with an estimated difference in $2 million over a 25-year career [84].

Having children can also impact salary. While never-married women in 2012 had almost closed the wage gap, earning 96% of what men earned, early work on the effect of motherhood on wages demonstrated that women with one child experience a 6% wage penalty and women with two or more children experience a 13% penalty [14]. Conversely, men do not incur such a penalty and may even have an increase in their wages after children, a phenomenon referred to as the "fatherhood bonus" [55]. There are several explanations offered for the motherhood gap penalty including interrupting their job or moving to part time to spend more time at home, accepting a "mother-friendly" job at the expense of a lower wage, being too tired from caring for children to maintain productivity at work, discrimination against mothers by employers, and the potential existence of an unmeasured factor associated with increased wages and lower likelihood of becoming a mother [15]. This "motherhood gap" is likely more significant in women in medicine. One study found that highly skilled women with higher wages experience more of a penalty than other groups, estimated up to 10% per child [29].

There is an incomplete understanding of the reason behind the gender-based differences in salary. While several theories have been posited, including differences in negotiation and family composition, the evidence to support these theories is mixed. One study looked for differences in starting salary across all medical specialties and found an adjusted difference of roughly $20,000 in 2017 [54]. The authors then set out to explain the differences in these starting salaries. Difference in medical specialty was responsible for the biggest portion of the difference in starting salary. However, after examining a wide set of variables, the authors were unable to find an explanation for 39% of the difference in starting salaries between men and women [54].

Correll et al., when examining reasons behind gender-based pay inequity, found that mothers are often viewed as less competent and less likely to want a promotion with the assumption that they would rather spend their time and energy at home [24]. The number of women in a field is responsible for up to 30% of the wage gap, whereas the combination of education and experience explained very little of this pay gap [80]. There have been other factors hypothesized to factor into the gender-based wage gap, including cognitive traits, noncognitive skills, preferences, attitude toward risk, differential rewarding of these traits on the basis of gender, and institution-specific policies, although these remain to be fully investigated [80].

Gender segregation—the predominance of a specific gender within a field—and devaluation, the concept that occupations dominated by women are devalued overtime [51, 66], are two other hypothesized reasons behind the pay gap. Once women begin to make up a significant proportion of specialty or field, the specialty rapidly experiences a shift toward a predominance of women. This "tipping effect" is hypothesized to be due to loss of occupational prestige once a field becomes saturated with women [63]. In medicine, increased segregation perpetuates this cycle. Fields dominated by women, such as pediatrics, are usually lower paid than those fields in which there is a predominance of men. Indeed, a longitudinal analysis of median salary in pediatrics found that the median salary for pediatricians in 1975 was 93% of the national physician salary when the field was 23% women [66]. Comparatively, in 2017 when the field was 63% women, the median income in pediatrics was 71% of the median physician income [66]. Thus, a feedback loop develops, especially given that men are more likely to rank salary higher than women when considering medical specialty choice [83]. Other proposed explanations for this troubling phenomenon include (1) equalizing differentials and (2) queueing. Equalizing differentials suggests that women select careers that require less investment and skill because they have other priorities, such as family obligations. However, when controlling for job characteristics in salary comparisons, the pay gap between men and women persists. Queueing posits that gender bias in hiring favors men, leaving women with less competitive, lower-paying jobs, while the devaluation theory suggests that work performed by women is systematically devalued, resulting in lower wages over time.

Gender Fair Pay Act

The Equal Pay Act of 1962 is an amendment to the Fair Labor Standards Act and makes it illegal to change wages on the basis of sex.[1] A stipulation of this act is that although job titles may be different, the jobs must be "substantially equal" between sexes. This act covers all aspects of compensation, including wages, bonuses, and benefits, among others. Later legislation includes the Lilly Ledbetter Fair Pay Act, which states that the time to file a lawsuit based on gender discrimination in salary resets with each paycheck, thus increasing the amount of time that a person can file suit for discrimination. This act also includes language around requiring documentation to justify all compensation and promotion decisions. However, the Lilly Ledbetter Fair Pay Act has not resulted in a significantly increased number of people filing suit for gender-based compensation claims [81]. Further legislative efforts to address the gender-based pay gap are necessary.

Salary Transparency

The lack of data regarding salaries within an organization or field is a significant barrier to reducing the salary gap [78]. One way that has been proposed to address the gender discrepancy in wages is salary transparency. A study of Canadian universities found that a law requiring disclosure of salaries of public sector employees reduced the gender-based gap in salaries by 20–40% [10]. Indeed, in settings where salaries are transparent, such as seen in unions and the federal workforce, there is a much lower wage gap when compared to other sectors [81]. Another benefit of salary transparency is enabling all new hires and current employee's data to use in salary negotiation. However, this benefits men more than women, as women who negotiate often face backlash and are less likely than men to be given a raise [6, 8]. Thus, while salary transparency is an important step in addressing the wage gap in medicine, it is not sufficient to fully address this issue alone.

Future Directions

Gender inequity persists in pediatrics despite gains in representation. Changes need to be made on multiple levels and domains to address this continued inequity. The state of inequity has been well-documented, and while continued efforts to track relevant metrics are critical to measuring progress, they are not sufficient. Conscious efforts to reduce barriers to entering the field, including ensuring sufficient numbers of role models, mentors, and sponsors, addressing pay inequity, expanding support

[1] The word "sex" is the term used in the legislation.

for parents, and combating bias at all stages of medical training and practice, are needed to address gender inequity. Accordingly, mitigation of unconscious bias in selection processes for leadership positions and promotion or tenure decisions remains paramount. Institutional efforts to systematically evaluate and mitigate salary inequity are needed to address the gender-based salary gaps. Finally, there is a critical need to support physicians of all genders who decide to start a family. This includes ensuring the availability of paid parental leave, lactation support, and assistance with costs of childcare. Gender inequity is a complex problem, and its pervasiveness both within society and our profession requires a multifaceted approach to create lasting, meaningful change. These efforts to promote equity may improve patient care, as there is data suggesting that women physicians are more likely to follow clinical guidelines [11], engage in more patient-centered conversations [71], and have better outcomes in certain populations when compared to physicians who are men [79, 82]. Further efforts to promote diversity will likely only serve to continue to improve care, and outcomes, for all children.

References

1. 2018 Survey of America's Physicians. 2018.
2. AAMC. 2015–2016 the state of women in academic medicine statistics. 2015.
3. AAMC. Table A-6: Age of Applicants to U. S. Medical Schools at Anticipated Matriculation by Sex and Race / Ethnicity, 2014–2015 through 2017–2018 Table A-6: Age of Applicants to U. S. Medical Schools at Anticipated Matriculation by Sex and Race / Ethnici. 2018
4. AAMC. 2018–2019 The state of women in academic medicine: Exploring pathways to equity. 2019
5. AMA Data: Physicians in Private Practice Continue to Decline | HealthLeaders Media. n.d. Retrieved December 15, 2021, from https://www.healthleadersmedia.com/clinical-care/ama-data-physicians-private-practice-continue-decline.
6. Amanatullah ET, Morris MW. Negotiating gender roles: gender differences in assertive negotiating are mediated by women's fear of backlash and attenuated when negotiating on behalf of others. J Pers Soc Psychol. 2010;98(2):256–67. https://doi.org/10.1037/a0017094.
7. Andriole DA, Whelan AJ, Jeffe DB. Characteristics and career intentions of the emerging MD/PhD workforce. JAMA. 2008;300(10):1165–73. https://doi.org/10.1001/jama.300.10.1165.
8. Artz B, Goodall AH, Oswald AJ. Do women ask? Ind Relat. 2018;57(4):611–36. https://doi.org/10.1111/irel.12214.
9. Association Cullof American Medical Colleges (AAMC). 2020 physician specialty report data highlights. 2020.
10. Baker M, Halberstam Y, Kroft K, Mas A, Messacar D. Pay transparency and the gender gap. National Bureau of Economic Research. Cambridge, MA; 2021.
11. Baumhäkel M, Müller U, Böhm M. Influence of gender of physicians and patients on guideline-recommended treatment of chronic heart failure in a cross-sectional study. Eur J Heart Fail. 2009;11(3):299–303. https://doi.org/10.1093/eurjhf/hfn041.
12. Bickel J, Rosenthal SL. Difficult issues in mentoring: recommendations on making the "undiscussable" discussable. Acad Med. 2011;86(10):1229–34. https://doi.org/10.1097/ACM.0b013e31822c0df7.
13. Bravender T, Selkie E, Sturza J, Martin DM, Griffith KA, Kaciroti N, Jagsi R. Association of salary differences between medical specialties with sex distribution. JAMA

Pediatr. 2021;175(5):524–5. American Medical Association. https://doi.org/10.1001/jamapediatrics.2020.5683

14. Budig MJ, England P. The wage penalty for motherhood author (s): Michelle J. Budig and Paula England published by: American Sociological Association stable. URL: http://www.jstor.org/stable/2657415. Accessed: 02-03-2016 03: 11 UTC Your use of the JSTOR archive indicates. 2001a; 66(2), 204–225.
15. Budig MJ, England P. The wage penalty for motherhood author (s): Michelle J. Budig and Paula England published by: American Sociological Association stable URL: http://www.jstor.org/stable/2657415 Accessed: 02-03-2016 03: 11 UTC Your use of the JSTOR archive indicates. 2001b;66(2), 204–225.
16. Byrne BJ, Katakam SK, Frintner MP, Cull WL. Early career experiences of pediatricians pursuing or not pursuing fellowship training. Pediatrics. 2015;136(4):672–9. https://doi.org/10.1542/peds.2014-3973.
17. Cain JM, Schulkin J, Parisi V, Power ML, Holzman GB, Williams S. Effects of perceptions and mentorship on pursuing a career in academic medicine in obstetrics and gynecology. Acad Med. 2001;76(6):628–34. https://doi.org/10.1097/00001888-200106000-00015.
18. Camacci ML, Ikpoh B, Lehman EB, Bowie E, Scott IU, Pantanelli SM, Ely A. Gender disparities among United States academic pediatric ophthalmologists: an analysis of publication productivity, academic rank, and NIH funding. J AAPOS. 2020;24(6):337.e1–6. https://doi.org/10.1016/j.jaapos.2020.06.013.
19. Carnes M, Bartels C, Isaac C, Kaatz A, Kolehmainen C. Why is John more likely to become department chair than Jennifer? Trans Am Clin Climatol Assoc. 2015;126:197–214.
20. Carr PL, Ash AS, Friedman RH, Scaramucci A, Barnett RC, Szalacha L, Palepu A, Moskowitz MA. Relation of family responsibilities and gender to the productivity and career satisfaction of medical faculty. Ann Intern Med. 1998;129(7):532–8. https://doi.org/10.7326/0003-4819-129-7-199810010-00004.
21. Catenaccio E, Rochlin JM, Simon HK. Differences in lifetime earning potential for pediatric subspecialists. Pediatrics. 2021a;147(4) https://doi.org/10.1542/peds.2020-027771.
22. Catenaccio E, Rochlin JM, Simon HK. Differences in lifetime earning potential between pediatric and adult physicians. Pediatrics. 2021b;148(2) https://doi.org/10.1542/peds.2021-051194.
23. Cooper M. For women leaders, likability and success hardly go hand-in-hand. Harvard Business Review, April 30th; 2013.
24. Correll SJ, Benard S, Paik I. Getting a job: is there a motherhood penalty? Am J Sociol. 2007;112(5):1297–338. https://doi.org/10.1086/511799.
25. Cull W, Caspary G, Olson L. Many pediatric residents seek and obtain part-time positions. Pediatrics. 2008;121(2):276–81. https://doi.org/10.1542/peds.2007-0311.
26. Cusimano MC, Baxter NN, Sutradhar R, Mcarthur E, Ray JG, Garg AX, Vigod S, Simpson AN. Delay of pregnancy among physicians vs nonphysicians supplemental content. JAMA Intern Med. 2021;181(7):905–12. https://doi.org/10.1001/jamainternmed.2021.1635.
27. Durfey, S. N. M., White, J., & Adashi, E. Y. (2021). Pregnancy and parenting in medical school: highlighting the need for data and support. Acad Med, 1259–1262. https://doi.org/10.1097/ACM.0000000000003988.
28. Edmunds LD, Ovseiko PV, Shepperd S, Greenhalgh T, Frith P, Roberts NW, Pololi LH, Buchan AM. Why do women choose or reject careers in academic medicine? A narrative review of empirical evidence. Lancet. 2016;388(10062):2948–58. https://doi.org/10.1016/S0140-6736(15)01091-0.
29. England P, Bearak J, Budig MJ, Hodges MJ. Do highly paid, highly skilled women experience the largest motherhood penalty? Am Sociol Rev. 2016;81(6):1161–89. https://doi.org/10.1177/0003122416673598.
30. Farkas AH, Bonifacino E, Turner R, Tilstra SA, Corbelli JA. Mentorship of women in academic medicine: a systematic review. J General Internal Med. 2019;34(7):1322–9. Springer New York LLC. https://doi.org/10.1007/s11606-019-04955-2

31. Fishman M, Williams WA, Goodman DM, Ross LF. Gender differences in the authorship of original research in Pediatric journals, 2001–2016. J Pediatr. 2017;191:244–249.e1. https://doi.org/10.1016/J.JPEDS.2017.08.044.
32. Fox G, Schwartz A, Hart KM. Work-family balance and academic advancement in medical schools. Acad Psychiatry. 2006;30(3):227–34. https://doi.org/10.1176/appi.ap.30.3.227.
33. Frank E. Career satisfaction of US women physicians. Arch Intern Med. 1999;159(13):1417. https://doi.org/10.1001/archinte.159.13.1417.
34. Frank E, Zhao Z, Sen S, Guille C. Gender disparities in work and parental status among early career physicians. JAMA Netw Open. 2019;2(8):–e198340. https://doi.org/10.1001/JAMANETWORKOPEN.2019.8340.
35. Freed GL, Moran LM, Van KD, Leslie LK. Current workforce of general pediatricians in the United States. Pediatrics. 2016;137(4) https://doi.org/10.1542/peds.2015-4242.
36. Freed GL, Moran LM, Van KD, Leslie LK. Current workforce of pediatric subspecialists in the United States. Pediatrics. 2017;139(5) https://doi.org/10.1542/peds.2016-3604.
37. Friedberg MW, Chen PG, Busum KRV, Aunon FM, Pham C, Caloyeras J, Mattke S, Pitchforth E, Quigley DD, Brook RH, Crosson FJ, Tutty M. RAND Study—Physician Satisfaction. 2013.
38. Frintner M, Mulvey H, Pletcher B,Olson L. Pediatric resident debt and career intentions. Pediatrics. 2013;131(2):312–8. https://doi.org/10.1542/peds.2012-0411.
39. Frintner MP, Cull WL, Byrne BJ, Freed GL, Katakam SK, Leslie LK, Miller AA, Starmer AJ, Olson LM. A longitudinal study of pediatricians early in their careers: places. Pediatrics. 2015;136(2):370–80. https://doi.org/10.1542/peds.2014-3972.
40. Frintner MP, Sisk B, Byrne BJ, Freed GL, Starmer AJ, Olson LM. Gender differences in earnings of early- and midcareer pediatricians. Pediatrics. 2019;144(4) https://doi.org/10.1542/peds.2018-3955.
41. Gerull K, Loe M, Seiler K, McAllister J, Salles A. Assessing gender bias in qualitative evaluations of surgical residents. The American Journal of Surgery. 2019;217(2):306–13. https://doi.org/10.1016/j.amjsurg.2018.09.029.
42. Gottlieb A.. Closing the Gender Pay Gap in Medicine | SpringerLink. Springer; 2021. https://link.springer.com/book/10.1007%2F978-3-030-51031-2.
43. Gottlieb AS, Jagsi R. Closing the gender pay gap in Medicine. N Engl J Med. 2021;NEJMp2114955 https://doi.org/10.1056/NEJMp2114955.
44. Harris MC, Marx J, Gallagher PR, Ludwig S. General vs subspecialty pediatrics: factors leading to residents' career decisions over a 12-year period. Arch Pediatr Adolesc Med. 2005;159(3):212–6). American Medical Association. https://doi.org/10.1001/archpedi.159.3.212.
45. Horowitz E, Randis TM, Samnaliev M, Savich R. Equity for women in medicine—neonatologists identify issues. J Perinatol. 2021;41(3):435–44. https://doi.org/10.1038/s41372-020-00897-4.
46. Isaac C, Chertoff J, Lee B, Carnes M. Do students' and authors' genders affect evaluations? A linguistic analysis of medical student performance evaluations. Acad Med. 2011;86(1):59–66. https://doi.org/10.1097/ACM.0b013e318200561d.
47. Jagsi R, Tarbell NJ, Weinstein DF. Becoming a doctor, starting a family—leaves of absence from graduate medical education. N Engl J Med. 2007;357(19):1889–91. https://doi.org/10.1056/nejmp078163.
48. Jolly S, Griffith KA, DeCastro R, Stewart A, Ubel P, Jagsi R. Gender differences in time spent on parenting and domestic responsibilities by high-achieving young physician-researchers. Ann Intern Med. 2014;160(5):344–53. https://doi.org/10.7326/m13-0974.
49. Klein R, Julian KA, Snyder ED, Koch J, Ufere NN, Volerman A, Vandenberg AE, Schaeffer S, Palamara K. Gender bias in resident assessment in graduate medical education: review of the literature. J General Internal Med. 2019;34(5):712–9. Springer New York LLC. https://doi.org/10.1007/s11606-019-04884-0.
50. Kolehmainen C, Brennan M, Filut M, Issac C, Carnes M. Afraid of Being Witchy with a 'B'": A Qualitative Study of How Gender Influences Residents' Experiences Leading

Cardiopulmonary Resuscitation. Acad Med. 2014;89(9):1276–81. https://doi.org/10.1097/ACM.0000000000000372.

51. Levanon A, England P, Paul Allison UOP. Occupational feminization and pay: assessing causal dynamics using 1950–2000 U.S. Census data. Soc Forces. 2009;88(2):865–91. https://doi.org/10.1353/sof.0.0264.
52. Levine R, Lin F, Kern D, Wright S, Carrese J. Stories from early-career women physicians who have left academic medicine: a qualitative study at a single institution. Acad Med 2011;86(6):752–8. https://doi.org/10.1097/ACM.0b013e318217e83b.
53. Levine R, Mechaber H, Reddy S, … D. C.-A., & 2013, undefined. "A good career choice for women": Female medical students' mentoring experiences: A multi-institutional qualitative study. Journals.Lww.Com. n.d.-b.
54. Lo Sasso AT, Armstrong D, Forte G, Gerber SE. Differences in starting pay for male and female physicians persist; explanations for the gender gap remain elusive. Health Aff. 2020;39(2):256–63. https://doi.org/10.1377/hlthaff.2019.00664.
55. Lundberg S, Rose E. Parenthood and the earnings of married men and women. Labour Econ. 2000;7(6):689–710. https://doi.org/10.1016/S0927-5371(00)00020-8.
56. Macy ML, Leslie LK, Turner A, Freed GL. Growth and changes in the pediatric medical subspecialty workforce pipeline. Pediatr Res. 2021;89(5):1297–303. https://doi.org/10.1038/s41390-020-01311-7.
57. Matulevicius S, Kho K, Reisch J, Open, H. Y.-J. Network, & 2021, undefined. Academic medicine faculty perceptions of work-life balance before and since the COVID-19 pandemic. Jamanetwork.Com. n.d.
58. McMurray JE, Linzer M, Konrad TR, Douglas J, Shugerman R, Nelson K. The work lives of women physicians: results from the physician work life study. J Gen Intern Med. 2000;15(6):372–80. https://doi.org/10.1046/j.1525-1497.2000.9908009.x.
59. McNamara MC, McNeil MA, Chang J. A pilot study exploring gender differences in residents' strategies for establishing mentoring relationships. Med Educ Online. 2008;13(1):4476. https://doi.org/10.3402/meo.v13i.4476.
60. Merritt Hawkins, & The Physicians Foundation. 2018 Survey of America's physicians practice patterns & perspectives. Physicians Foundation; 2018. p. 1–82.
61. Morales-Lemieux K. How compensation is determined and potential pitfalls for pay equity. In: Gotttlieb A, editor. Closing the gender pay gap in medicine: a roadmap for healthcare organizations and the women physicians who work for them. Springer; 2021. p. 17–28. https://doi.org/10.4018/978-1-5225-9599-1.ch008.
62. O'Meara KA, Kuvaeva A, Nyunt G, Waugaman C, Jackson R. Asked more often: gender differences in faculty workload in research universities and the work interactions that shape them. Am Educ Res J. 2017;54(6):1154–86. https://doi.org/10.3102/0002831217716767.
63. Pan J. Gender segregation in occupations: the role of tipping and social interactions. J Labor Econ. 2015;33(2):365–408. https://doi.org/10.1086/678518.
64. Pediatrics AB of. Yearly growth in general pediatrics residents by demographics and program characteristics. n.d. Retrieved January 6, 2022, from https://www.abp.org/content/yearly-growth-general-pediatrics-residents-demographics-and-program-characteristics.
65. Pediatrics, T. A. B. of. The American Board of Pediatrics, Research Department. 2021.
66. Pelley E, Carnes M. When a specialty becomes "women's work": trends in and implications of specialty gender segregation in Medicine. Acad Med. 2020;95(10):1499–506. https://doi.org/10.1097/ACM.0000000000003555.
67. Perumalswami CR, Takenoshita S, Tanabe A, Kanda R, Hiraike H, Okinaga H, Jagsi R, Nomura K. Workplace resources, mentorship, and burnout in early career physician-scientists: a cross sectional study in Japan. BMC Med Educ. 2020;20(1):1–10. https://doi.org/10.1186/s12909-020-02072-x.
68. Richter KP, Clark L, Wick JA, Cruvinel E, Durham D, Shaw P, Shih GH, Befort CA, Simari RD. Women physicians and promotion in academic Medicine. N Engl J Med. 2020;383(22):2148–57. https://doi.org/10.1056/nejmsa1916935.

69. Ross DA, Boatright D, Nunez-Smith M, Jordan A, Chekroud A, Moore EZ. Differences in words used to describe racial and gender groups in medical student performance evaluations. PLoS One. 2017;12(8) https://doi.org/10.1371/journal.pone.0181659.
70. Rotbart HA, McMillen D, Taussig H, Daniels SR. Assessing gender equity in a large academic Department of Pediatrics. Acad Med. 2012;87(1):98–104. https://doi.org/10.1097/ACM.0b013e31823be028.
71. Roter DL, Hall JA, Aoki Y. Physician gender effects in medical communication: a meta-analytic review. J Am Med Assoc. 2002;288(6):756–64. https://doi.org/10.1001/jama.288.6.756.
72. Schor NF. The decanal divide. Acad Med. 2018;93(2):237–40. https://doi.org/10.1097/ACM.0000000000001863.
73. Silver JK, Poorman JA, Reilly JM, Spector ND, Goldstein R, Zafonte RD. Assessment of women physicians among authors of perspective-type articles published in high-impact Pediatric journals. JAMA Netw Open. 2018;1(3):e180802. https://doi.org/10.1001/jamanetworkopen.2018.0802.
74. Spector ND, Asante PA, Marcelin JR, Poorman JA, Larson AR, Salles A, Oxentenko AS, Silver JK. Women in pediatrics: Progress, barriers, and opportunities for equity, diversity, and inclusion. Pediatrics. 2019;144(5) https://doi.org/10.1542/peds.2019-2149.
75. Spencer SJ, Logel C, Davies PG. Stereotype threat. Annu Rev Psychol. 2016;67:415–37. https://doi.org/10.1146/annurev-psych-073115-103235.
76. Starmer AJ, Frintner MP, Matos K, Somberg C, Freed G, Byrne BJ. Gender discrepancies related to pediatrician work-life balance and household responsibilities. Pediatrics. 2019;144(4) https://doi.org/10.1542/peds.2018-2926.
77. Stentz NC, Griffith KA, Perkins E, Jones RD, Jagsi R. Fertility and childbearing among American female physicians. J Women's Health. 2016;25(10):1059–65. https://doi.org/10.1089/jwh.2015.5638.
78. Trotter RG, Zacur SR, Stickney LT. The new age of pay transparency. Bus Horiz. 2017;60(4):529–39. https://doi.org/10.1016/j.bushor.2017.03.011.
79. Tsugawa Y, Jena AB, Figueroa JF, Orav EJ, Blumenthal DM, Jha AK. Comparison of hospital mortality and readmission rates for medicare patients treated by male vs female physicians. JAMA Intern Med. 2017;177(2):206–13. https://doi.org/10.1001/jamainternmed.2016.7875.
80. United WB, Chakravorty A, Murdoch J, Nisar H. Gender-based pay disparity study. 2019.
81. Wade M, Fiorentino S. Gender pay inequality: an examination of the Lilly Ledbetter fair pay act six years later. Adv Women Leadersh. 2017;37:29–36.
82. Wallis CJ, Ravi B, Coburn N, Nam RK, Detsky AS, Satkunasivam R. Comparison of postoperative outcomes among patients treated by male and female surgeons: a population based matched cohort study. BMJ (Online). 2017;359 https://doi.org/10.1136/bmj.j4366.
83. West CP, Drefahl MM, Popkave C, Kolars JC. Internal medicine resident self-report of factors associated with career decisions. J Gen Intern Med. 2009;24(8):946–9. https://doi.org/10.1007/s11606-009-1039-0.
84. Whaley CM, Koo T, Arora VM, Ganguli I, Gross N, Jena AB. Female physicians earn an estimated $2 million less than male physicians over a simulated 40-year career. Health Aff. 2021;40(12):1856–64. https://doi.org/10.1377/hlthaff.2021.00461.

Chapter 4
Leadership in Pediatrics

Kelsey Logan and Archana Chatterjee

Introduction

"You can't be what you can't see." This sentence, attributed to the American activist Marian Wright Edelman, is commonly used to describe the barrier of not being able to see someone like yourself achieve success or attain a leadership position. Many girls can see women as pediatricians, as this generation likely has a woman for a primary care physician. In 2019, 64.3% of active physicians in pediatrics were women [10]. Can they see a woman in leadership, though?

In its "Blueprint for Action: Visioning Summit on the Future of the Workforce in Pediatrics" [39], the Federation of Pediatric Organizations noted that "Changes have occurred in education and training, clinical practice, research, and leadership that have resulted in the transformation of the profession of pediatrics, resulting in increasing workforce and leadership diversity and gender equity." One of the priorities focused on in this blueprint was "Acknowledge the impact that the increasing proportion of women has on the field of pediatrics." This resulted in a vision statement that the profession be strengthened by optimizing "expertise, leadership, and diversity in a changing pediatric workforce." Fair pay, representation, and promotion based on meritocracy make sense to us; however, they are not practiced in the vast majority of medicine as of 2021. We delve into the scope of the leadership gap and how to resolve it in this chapter.

K. Logan (✉)
Division of Sports Medicine, Cincinnati Children's Hospital Medical Center, University of Cincinnati College of Medicine, Cincinnati, OH, USA
e-mail: Kelsey.logan@cchmc.org

A. Chatterjee
Rosalind Franklin University of Medicine and Science, Chicago Medical School, North Chicago, IL, USA
e-mail: Archana.chatterjee@rosalindfranklin.edu

N. D. Spector et al. (eds.), *Women in Pediatrics*,
https://doi.org/10.1007/978-3-030-98222-5_4

The Importance of Women in Leadership

Women report less control than men on the daily demands of a physician's life: managing clinic and office schedules and patient volume and controlling workplace issues [32]. Women have also been shown to be at risk for burnout when they lack power in the workplace and control over their work schedule [32]. From a practical standpoint, having women in leadership could help women who are not in positions of power improve their lives. The effect of having someone in leadership who can understand the cultural norms, pressures, and experiences of women cannot be overestimated. Of course, this is most likely to be a woman, but a man certainly can play the same role. Indeed, we are counting on men to play this role.

In the business world, having women in leadership has been associated with improved financial performance, with an average 15% profitability increase for those firms going to 30% women in corporate leadership [35]. There is also improved equity for female executives and improved practices for the entire workforce, such as paternity leave [36]. McKinsey & Company found that companies highest in "gender diversity on their executive teams are 21% more likely than other firms to report above-average profitability" [31]. Theories for this effect include "increased skill diversity within top management, which increases effectiveness in monitoring staff performance, and less gender discrimination through the management ranks, which helps to recruit, promote, and retain talent" [35].

Medical and professional outcomes may also be better with a woman's influence [9]. For hospitalists, readmission and in-hospital mortality rates are lower for patients who have female physicians [9, 42]. Particularly interesting is a 2018 study of mortality in heart attack patients, shown to be higher in female patients treated by a male physician. Mortality rates decreased "when male physicians practice(d) with more female colleagues" [24].

Fairness

Gender equality in pediatric leadership is a "matter of fairness and social justice" [40]. In 2019, 64.3% of active pediatricians in the USA were women [10], and 72.4% of pediatric residents and fellows were women [2]. Despite the majority of pediatricians being women, women held only 26.2% (41 of 149) of Pediatric Department Chair positions in 2018 [41].

The Her Time is Now Campaign [26] emphasizes focusing on and discussing gatekeeping in career advancement in academic medicine "through the combined lens of how ethical conduct and financial support intersect." This is an important document with candid assessments of gender bias and suggestions for fairness/gender equity. The effect of intersectionality is also addressed in the report and should be acknowledged as a barrier particularly for women from minoritized backgrounds attaining leadership positions. The authors note that for their 2020 report, "many of the same issues apply to women working in all healthcare settings and in fields beyond medicine." Highlighted in the report is the combination of structural and institutional gender bias that impairs career advancement at every level. This impairment makes the timeline for promotion so lengthy that women are at risk for not being promoted, even by the time they retire.

As a mother with a 9-year-old daughter, I (Logan) am concerned about her likelihood for success in the medical or corporate world, should the current environment not change. I wonder if she will carry the same anxiety I have into rooms full of men making decisions, with me being the only woman. I wonder if she will be interrupted when she has the courage to voice an idea, or if she will be encouraged and supported by a woman leader to speak up.

I too (Chatterjee) am a mother, and my daughter is currently a medical student. Unfortunately, I see her face some of the same sexism, discrimination, and misogyny that I did a generation ago. I do believe that she is empowered through her education and life experiences thus far to be able to speak up and bring about needed change, but it is still an uphill task. There is much work to be done to reduce (and ideally, eliminate) the biases against women in medicine that persist despite efforts to remove them.

Scope of the Issue

The gaps between income, promotion, and leadership positions between men and women discussed in this chapter have persisted even though the "pipeline" of women is more than sufficient for gender parity, especially in pediatrics [41]. When discussing the status of women in pediatric leadership, the significance of cultural bias against women cannot be ignored. The leadership status of women in pediatrics follows what we understand about the status of women overall in our male-dominated leadership culture.

There is extensive research illustrating the bias against women in medicine and science. For example, a 2012 study of 127 academic science faculty showed the faculty (men and women) rated a male applicant for a manager position as "significantly more competent and hirable than the (identical) female applicant" [33]. In this same study, faculty offered less career mentoring and smaller salaries to women, even as they reported liking the female applicants more than the male applicants. The authors concluded that this inequity could shape the self-efficacy, goal-setting, and ultimate career trajectory of women in scientific fields.

The Pay Gap

In 2021, the income gap between men and women physicians is well documented, with studies reporting 16–37% difference, with men making more money than women [1]. The gender pay gap for physicians is one of the largest in the USA, with women physicians earning "75 cents on the dollar compared with their male counterparts" [34]. This mirrors the income gap in society as a whole, in which women are paid 82 cents for every dollar paid to men, for the same work [7]. In their discussion of gender income gaps in all medical specialties, the authors of a manuscript detailing results of the Physician Work Life Study noted that "slower promotion to positions of leadership" may contribute to this income gap. They theorized that the study's results, showing that differences exist between men and women in "patient mix, time pressure in patient visits, income, control of daily work life, and burnout" contribute to leadership and income gaps [32]. Women typically do more work-related citizenship tasks (and feel less in control of their obligation to these tasks), such as acting as a required representative, serving on committees, and working in recruitment efforts. This work, which has been proposed as a "tax" that disproportionately effects women, may impair their compensation and promotion to leadership [8].

Inequity in wages is theorized to occur in part due to occupational segregation, with work done by women systemically undervalued [7]. Professions dominated by women have lower incomes, and women are overrepresented in low-wage fields [23]. Pelley and Carnes have written about the pattern known as "tipping" – once a certain number of women enter a profession that was previously dominated by men, that profession experiences a rapid decline of men entering the profession (e.g., bank tellers, secretaries, and teachers). In medicine, this is particularly felt in pediatrics and obstetrics-gynecology, the two most women-predominant specialties, where salary relative to the average physician has declined ~20% in four decades [37].

"The Motherhood Penalty" also contributes to the pay gap, in which lower salaries and fewer promotions are offered to women who have children than to women without children. Coupled with the fact that "fathers make 119% of what men without children earn," the so-called "Fatherhood Bonus," these effects "result in women with children earning only 73% of what fathers earn" [7].

The Promotion and Leadership Gaps

In academic medicine, the Association of American Medical Colleges (AAMC) published 2014 statistics on female leadership, with women comprising 21% of full professors, 15% of department chairs, and 16% of deans [29]. Data from the 2018 to 2019 AAMC survey showed that "the number of women deans increased by about one each year, on average" from 2013 to 2018, with 18% of medical school deans being women in 2018 [5]. The promotion gap persists but is slowly improving, with women comprising 25% of full professors per the 2018–2019 AAMC data; still, the majority of women faculty remain at the lowermost rank of instructor (58%) [5]. Interestingly, 26.2% of pediatric chairs being women in 2018 [41] and 2019 data showing that less than 20% of academic medicine department chairs are women are very similar to the proportion of women who are deans [5, 12]. For women of color, this "leaky pipeline" is worse; 2018–2019 AAMC data show that underrepresented in medicine women "made up 15% of women chairs in basic science and clinical science departments" [5]. To address this issue, the AAMC Group on Women in Medicine and Science has developed toolkits for education and intervention in their "Strategies for Advancing the Careers of Women of Color in Academic Medicine" [3].

Leadership in medical societies has been deemed one of the crucial areas to address, as this leadership is influential in setting policy and changing pediatric practice. Medical societies have been identified as a "gatekeeper" to career advancement in academic medicine by the Her Time is Now Campaign ("Her Time is Now Report. Version 2"). The specialty of pediatrics struggles to equitably represent women in senior leadership, with only 37.5% (three of eight) of president-equivalent positions being held by women. However, there are signs that this could change, as women comprised 54.5% of pediatric society board positions in 2019 [27, 41].

Outside medicine, a 2014 sample of 21,980 firms in 91 countries was studied to quantify female leadership. Less than 5% of organizations had a female CEO and over half had no female "C-suite" members [36]. In 2021, the European Union (EU) reported that women held 7.8% of Board Chair and 8.2% of CEO positions in the largest publicly listed companies in the EU. Less than 29% of board members in those companies are women [20].

The Queen Bee Phenomenon

One argument for women's leadership assumes that women leaders support and grow other women leaders, eventually resulting in a gender-equitable leadership structure. However, when women are in organizations where leadership is male-dominated, evidence shows that the same hierarchical structure is more likely reinforced than changed. Even more discouraging is that "queen bees" in organizational structures hold other women back, instead of supporting them in advancement opportunities. Derks et al. discussed the "queen bee" as a woman "who pursue(s) individual success in male dominated-work settings by adjusting to the masculine culture and by distancing (herself) from other women" [17]. Because of the cultural bias against them and their lower perceived gender role, women who adopt a "queen bee"-type practice are likely doing so in an attempt to resolve their personal leadership disadvantage. Particularly in emphasizing the typically male-associated characteristics of leadership, women may feel the need to simulate their male colleagues in order to succeed. Further research has shown that women in leadership tend to support each other (and quotas) at the same organizational hierarchical level but see themselves as different, having sacrificed more, than junior women in the organization [21]. This attitude of perceiving great sacrifice to rise in leadership may make it less likely for a senior woman to support a junior woman who she does not see as having the same drive to succeed.

Promising Practices: Changing the Status Quo

If nothing changes, it has been estimated that it may take 50 years to reach gender parity in medical leadership [12]! The COVID-19 pandemic in 2020, with the associated job losses and inequities disproportionately affecting women, is seen as further threatening even that shocking forecast [4]. The importance of career development for women has become magnified: men and women leaders, as the change-makers of organizations, must elevate gender equity issues for fair treatment, pay, and promotion to leadership. These topics include the range of issues discussed in this and other chapters of this book. Additionally, there are practical solutions that the pandemic has illuminated and leaders can implement, such as normalizing conversations around life-work integration, developing and supporting peer professional networks, providing flexible work and teaching options, and alleviating child and family care stresses [28, 34].

Changing the status quo involves tactics complementary to those presented below and are included in other chapters of this book. As an example, suggested topics/questions to address are listed in Table 4.1.

What Men in Leadership in Pediatrics Can Do

Notice that this section comes before the "What Women in Leadership in Pediatrics Can Do" and the "What Women Can Do" sections. This is purposeful, as we must not demand that women make/lead the changes needed to combat the bias and unfair practices against them alone or primarily. It is neither practical nor fair to ask this.

Intentional change is needed among male leaders in pediatric healthcare organizations, medical societies, medical journals, and funding organizations [13]. The evidence behind gender inequity across the breadth of pediatrics is clear; ignorance about the problem or disregarding it is not acceptable. Men in positions of power can and should change the status quo by educating themselves and their peers, measuring the problem in their organization, and using metrics to resolve it. Use of the

Table 4.1 Questions for leaders in academic medicine

What else can be done in academic medicine to ensure fair pay for women?
What can academic institutions (i.e., employers) do to ensure that women faculty are promoted fairly to assistant, associate, and full professor?
What can academic institutions do to ensure that women's time and effort in diversity, equity, and inclusion work is financially supported and given high priority for academic promotion?
What can academic institutions do to ensure that all of their faculty have equitable opportunities at medical societies?

This text was adapted with permission from Her Time is Now Report. Version 2. Published September 1, 2020. Available at https://sheleadshealthcare.com/.

Her Time is Now Report ("Her Time is Now Report. Version 2") to highlight gender inequity issues and pose questions leaders can ask themselves and their institution can be a good starting place. On an individual level, sponsoring women, in addition to mentoring them, results in purposeful, mindful promotion.

Some men will lead by example and encourage their fellow leaders to do the same. These voices are crucial and result in positive peer pressure that can be very influential. For example, at the 2021 AAMC Spring Council of Deans meeting, Dr. Francis Collins, Director of the National Institutes of Health, spoke about his practice with panels he is asked to participate in. He asks about other participants on the panel, and if no women are included, refuses the invitation. He said he does not want to be part of a "Manel" (a panel of experts that consists of men only) and that when organizers look for participants with gender diversity in mind, they usually find highly qualified people (F. Collins, personal communication, May 7, 2021).

What Women in Pediatrics Leadership Can Do

Alongside men in leadership positions, women leaders must be intentional about promoting leadership skill development among women in the pediatric workforce. Leadership training for women physicians must be part of institutional planning and metrics, and leaders must be held accountable for it. Some examples of highly effective leadership training programs are listed in Table 4.2.

Budgetary support of women for these types of programs, and others, is necessary, as is the time needed to participate. Leaders can and should provide this.

We know that sponsorship is crucial for junior employee and faculty success; women leaders are essential in this role, and the tenets of sponsorship are noted in the preceding paragraph. However, combating the "queen bee" phenomenon is challenging when women remain in male-dominated organizations, especially if they

Table 4.2 Examples of leadership training programs (many focused specifically on developing women leaders)

The Executive Leadership in Academic Medicine (ELAM) program [19] (longitudinal program)
Association of American Medical Colleges (AAMC) mid-career women faculty leadership development seminar [6]
AAMC early career women faculty leadership development seminar
AAMC minority faculty leadership development seminar
Women's Wellness through Equity and Leadership [43] collaborative [38]
Association of Medical School Pediatric Department Chairs (AMSPDC) Pediatric leadership development program [11]
Harvard Medical School career advancement and leadership skills for women in healthcare program
ADVANCE gender equity symposium
Women in Medicine summit
FemInPEM conference

see themselves as having sacrificed significantly for leadership opportunities. Research shows that "the tendency of successful women to resist affirmative action programs stems from their own career experiences" [21]. The intersection of work and family stress, lack of promotion and salary fairness, and the existing cultural and organizational gender bias make rising to positions of leadership seem daunting. Making the climb to leadership less stressful for women who are earlier in their careers can mitigate this and is part of this book's focus.

The impact of having women leaders for the authors has been immense. For one author (Chatterjee), having the support of a woman Provost and President/CEO helped her transition to her role as the first woman Dean and person of color to lead her medical school. Faced with the triple challenges of the pandemic, racial justice issues, and a looming accreditation visit, Dr. Chatterjee stated: "I had shattered a glass ceiling. I should have expected some of the shards to fall on me. If I backed out in this time of crisis, it would perhaps jeopardize the chance for other women who might follow in my footsteps. It was a heavy burden to bear, but one of my own choosing. It was also a great privilege that I did not feel I could relinquish lightly" [16]. For one author (Logan), having a woman Chair of Pediatrics "helped normalize work-life balance stress and provided a sounding board for how to navigate the pressures of being a Division Director while mothering three young children." Equally valuable was the Chair's intentionality in discussing promotion and how to achieve it. In addition, the sponsorship of women leaders in the Office of Academic Affairs and Career Development led to leadership training opportunities invaluable to career progression.

As a Department Chair, Dr. Chatterjee encouraged many women faculty members to aspire to leadership positions. One such faculty member was hesitant to take on leadership roles due to her family responsibilities. Dr. Chatterjee encouraged her to attend the AAMC Mid-Career Women Faculty Leadership Development Seminar [6]. Upon her return from the seminar, the faculty member took on the role of Division Chief. When a subsequent decanal position opened up, she asked Dr. Chatterjee if she should apply for it. With Dr. Chatterjee's encouragement and support, she was appointed as an Assistant Dean. This is an example of the value of sponsorship and the empowerment of women pediatricians as self-advocates.

What Institutions Can Do

It is established that gender bias is pervasive and present as "woven into the organization's culture" [30]. The result is that leadership decisions are based on bias and not on merit. As noted in the introduction to this chapter, this can lead to the promotion of women occurring at a slow rate or not at all.

The programs mentioned above are very selective. To achieve gender leadership equity in pediatrics, more women than can be served by high-level programming must have training that enables them to negotiate their work life and income, advocate for themselves for promotion and leadership training, and influence decision-making. Mid-career support for women, in particular, can get women to the leadership positions shown to improve organizational performance [35]. Institutions that are offering career training sessions or programming for women physicians, whether it be for early-, mid-, or late-career physicians, must keep metrics on participant career trajectory and promotion to leadership positions. By publishing results of those programs, "Best Practices" can be developed, evolved, and spread to other institutions. These metrics can be used to develop scorecards for institutional success on gender equity, further enhancing Best Practices.

Transparency of these metrics, and how institutions compare on gender equity success, is important in attracting and sustaining a workforce of women across all specialties. The BeEthical Campaign [13] supports this approach, calling on leaders to "document and correct workforce disparities in an efficient and effective manner" by using longitudinal data analysis and transparency of "process, analysis, and results." BeEthical has published proposed metrics for leaders and a process for leaders to use those metrics in evaluating gender equity [13]. These metrics include research funding and salary support, administrative time, and committee work that partially account for promotion inequity and often go underrecognized [12]. The promotion gap can be addressed in part by "adopting flexible promotion and advancement criteria, including promotion tracks that reflect the wide range of responsibilities and unique contributions of female physicians" [1].

Male dominance in medical leadership has become the default position; this must be challenged by a combination of culture change, reduction in and eventually, elimination of implicit biases toward women, and policies that support gender equity. "Subtle sexism" is a complicated problem that extends from our cultural beliefs and existing workplace systems; "subtle bias may make it challenging for women to ascend organizational hierarchies even in the absence of overt discrimination" [18]. There is some evidence that intentional work, even if brief, in addressing gender bias may improve outcomes and actions to promote gender equity. Carnes et al. conducted intervention over a 2.5-hour workshop for faculty at an academic medical center, focused on "gender bias-habit changing," that significantly improved survey scores on gender bias topics that support women in their career advancement [15].

Suggested policy changes include term limits for leaders [12] and mandated representation on corporate boards and political leadership roles [20, 36]. As the presence of women on boards may improve the "pipeline" for leadership roles in the organization, quotas have been proposed and used in some cases to support gender diversity [35]. Research shows that women who announce a pregnancy or are returning from maternity leave "described being passed over for leadership roles in favor of colleagues perceived as less qualified"; possible mitigating measures are to change "policies that exclude part time physicians from leadership roles" [25].

What Women Pediatricians Can Do

Awareness of gender-based leadership barriers is important for all women to have. For example, being able to recognize that "women leaders being mistaken for support staff" is a sign that the organizational culture associates leadership with masculinity or that "women having to learn how to lead on their own without a mentor" is an organizational lack of mentoring problem. Diehl et al. [18] provide more examples of gender-based leadership barriers and a Gender Bias Scale that are helpful to raise awareness of potential bias and that can be used to help organizations understand where issues lie, from the perspective of the women in the organization.

Women preparing for leadership will need the support of mentors and sponsors, both men and women. Gaining that support, for most, requires intentional skill development. While some women may naturally advocate for themselves, others find this difficult. Whether formally, such as in a course, or informally by individual learning/networking, skill development is needed. Table 4.3 lists topics that have been helpful to the authors but is not necessarily comprehensive:

One author (Logan) has found that a combination of individual learning to address some topics in depth (e.g., learning to say no and fighting imposter syndrome) and proactively asking about opportunities available for formal education is helpful. Engaging men as allies to help in challenging situations, and finding a peer group of women for support, has also been valuable. For Dr. Logan: "Advocating for myself and my leadership goals means (1) saying 'no' to anything that is not aligned with my goals, (2) discontinuing work that does not contribute to the institutional or professional mission, (3) it's ok to push back, and (4) it's ok to seek and accept help." For Dr. Chatterjee, being open to opportunities, selecting those aligned with her values and goals, and seeking the advice of mentors and sponsors were all helpful in her career development.

Table 4.3 Topics for skill development

"Graceful self-promotion" – Speaking about oneself and one's accomplishments with style and confidence
Improving professional visibility
Building a professional network
Sponsorship
Transforming conflict into positive change
Role transition
Negotiating successfully
Unconscious bias
Strategic planning
Developing financial savvy
Learning how to (and when to) say no
Wellness

What Else Needs to Be Done?

Legal and Societal Actions

Governmental action may be needed to accelerate the incredibly slow progress toward gender parity. In business, representation of women on corporate boards is mandated in several countries (e.g., France, Spain, Norway), and reporting on gender diversity and improvement is required of companies with more than 300 employees in Japan [31]. India requires that 33% of local government roles be held by women [31].

Pay equity laws have been passed in almost every state in the USA, but either the lack of consistent enforcement or limited scope makes them less effective than they could be [7]. In addition, banning private employer access to salary history has resulted in increased wages when women change jobs [14]; this is a change that could be widened to cover both public and private organizations in all states.

Supportive actions to advance women in leadership include increased education and training, mentoring and sponsorship, flexibility in work practices, and adequate and affordable child care options [7].

Challenging the Future

For gender parity in leadership to occur, we must start at the beginning of women pediatricians' careers. There is much work to do, as they start already behind men. Early to mid-career women pediatricians earn 76–94% of what male pediatricians do [22]. By mid-career, the inequities are compounded. In their manuscript "Is Academic Medicine Making Mid-Career Women Physicians Invisible?", Lewiss et al. conclude that women in mid-career "are at continued risk of being made invisible" due to lack of equal reward for accomplishments and that "It is especially important for the academic community to recognize that women…continue to lose ground at this juncture and are unable to be equitably represented at all levels of medicine including top leadership positions" [30]. Ultimately, this leads to the gaps in promotion and leadership we currently have.

But, we have hope! We are close to a critical mass of women in pediatric leadership positions and know more about how to develop and support women leaders. We can combine this with challenging current pay structures and lack of transparency. Implementing gender parity metrics and making those transparent to employees is a step that layers upon the prior steps and supports leadership opportunities for women. To improve the health of pediatrics as a specialty, it is time for us to make changes needed to achieve leadership equity that represents the stake women have in the specialty.

References

1. Achieving gender equity in physician compensation and career advancement: a position paper of the American College of Physicians. Ann Intern Med. 2018;168(10):721–3. https://doi.org/10.7326/m17-3438%m29710100.
2. American Association of Medical Colleges. 2019 physician specialty data report: Table 2.2 Number and Percentage of ACGME Residents and Fellows by Sex and Specialty, 2019. Retrieved from https://www.aamc.org/data-reports/interactive-data/acgme-residents-and-fellows-sex-and-specialty-2019.
3. American Association of Medical Colleges. Diversity and Inclusion: Women Faculty of Color Toolkits. Retrieved from https://www.aamc.org/professional-development/affinity-groups/gwims/women-of-color-initiative-toolkits.
4. American Association of Medical Colleges. How COVID-19 threatens the careers of women in medicine. November 12, 2020. Retrieved from https://www.aamc.org/news-insights/how-covid-19-threatens-careers-women-medicine#:~:text=More%20than%2020%20women%20physicians,%2C%20versus%2036%25%20of%20men.
5. American Association of Medical Colleges. The State of Women in Academic Medicine 2018-19: Exploring Pathways to Equity. Retrieved from https://store.aamc.org/downloadable/download/sample/sample_id/330/.
6. American Association of Medical Colleges: Mid-Career Women Faculty Leadership Development Seminar. Retrieved from https://www.aamc.org/professional-development/leadership-development/midwims.
7. American Association of University Women. The simple truth about the gender pay gap. 2020. Retrieved from https://www.aauw.org/app/uploads/2020/12/SimpleTruth_2.1.pdf.
8. Armijo PR, Silver JK, Larson AR, Asante P, Shillcutt S. Citizenship tasks and women physicians: additional woman tax in academic Medicine? J Womens Health (Larchmt). 2020; https://doi.org/10.1089/jwh.2020.8482.
9. Asgari MM, Carr PL, Bates CK. Closing the gender wage gap and achieving professional equity in Medicine. JAMA. 2019;321(17):1665–6. https://doi.org/10.1001/jama.2019.4168.
10. Association of American Medical Colleges. Number and Percentage of Active Physicians by Sex and Specialty, 2019; Table 1.3. Retrieved from https://www.aamc.org/data-reports/workforce/interactive-data/active-physicians-sex-and-specialty-2019.
11. Association of Medical School Pediatric Department Chairs, I. Retrieved from https://amspdc.org/pldp/.
12. Beeler WH, Mangurian C, Jagsi R. Unplugging the pipeline – a call for term limits in academic Medicine. N Engl J Med. 2019;381(16):1508–11. https://doi.org/10.1056/NEJMp1906832.
13. BeEthical: A Call to Healthcare Leaders: Ending Gender Workforce Disparities is an Ethical Imperative, v4. (Published September 17, 2018). Retrieved from https://sheleadshealthcare.com/wp-content/uploads/2018/09/Be-Ethical-Campaign.pdf.
14. Bessen JE a. M., Chen and Denk, Erich, Perpetuating Inequality: What Salary History Bans Reveal About Wages (June 2020). Retrieved from SSRN: https://ssrn.com/abstract=3628729 or https://doi.org/10.2139/ssrn.3628729.
15. Carnes M, Devine PG, Baier Manwell L, Byars-Winston A, Fine E, Ford CE, Sheridan J. The effect of an intervention to break the gender bias habit for faculty at one institution: a cluster randomized, controlled trial. Acad Med. 2015;90(2):221–30. https://doi.org/10.1097/acm.0000000000000552.
16. Chatterjee A. Lessons Learned – Women Dean Leaders in the US session. 2021, March 26, 2021. Paper presented at the AMWA Leads 2021.
17. Derks B, Laar C, Ellemers N. The queen bee phenomenon: why women leaders distance themselves from junior women. Leadersh Q. 2016;27:456–69. https://doi.org/10.1016/j.leaqua.2015.12.007.

18. Diehl A, Stephenson A, Dzubinski L, Wang D. Measuring the invisible: development and multi-industry validation of the gender bias scale for women leaders. Human Res Develop Quarter. 2020;32(2):225–9.
19. Drexel University Collge of Medicine: Executive Leadership in Academic Medicine. About ELAM. Retrieved from https://drexel.edu/medicine/academics/womens-health-and-leadership/elam/about-elam/.
20. European Commission. Achieving gender balance in decision-making. Retrieved from https://ec.europa.eu/info/policies/justice-and-fundamental-rights/gender-equality/equality-between-women-and-men-decision-making/achieving-gender-balance-decision-making_en.
21. Faniko K, Ellemers N, Derks B, Lorenzi-Cioldi F. Nothing changes, really: why women who break through the glass ceiling end up reinforcing it. Pers Social Psychol Bull. 2017;43(5):638–51. https://doi.org/10.1177/0146167217695551.
22. Frintner MP, Sisk B, Byrne BJ, Freed GL, Starmer AJ, Olson LM. Gender differences in earnings of early- and midcareer pediatricians. Pediatrics. 2019;144(4) https://doi.org/10.1542/peds.2018-3955.
23. Gottlieb ASE. Closing the gender pay gap in medicine. Switzerland, AG: Springer Nature; 2021.
24. Greenwood BN, Carnahan S, Huang L. Patient-physician gender concordance and increased mortality among female heart attack patients. Proc Natl Acad Sci U S A. 2018;115(34):8569–74. https://doi.org/10.1073/pnas.1800097115.
25. Halley MC, Rustagi AS, Torres JS, Linos E, Plaut V, Mangurian C, Linos E. Physician mothers' experience of workplace discrimination: a qualitative analysis. BMJ. 2018;363:k4926.
26. Her Time is Now Report. Version 2. (Published September 1, 2020.). Retrieved from https://sheleadshealthcare.com/.
27. Jagsi R, Means O, Lautenberger D, Jones RD, Griffith KA, Flotte TR, Chatterjee A. Women's representation among members and leaders of national medical specialty societies. Acad Med. 2020;95(7):1043–9.
28. Kreeger PK, Brock A, Gibbs HC, Grande-Allen KJ, Huang AH, Masters KS, Servoss SL. Ten simple rules for women principal investigators during a pandemic. PLoS Comput Biol. 2020;16(10):–e1008370. https://doi.org/10.1371/journal.pcbi.1008370.
29. Lautenberger DM, Dandar VM, Raezer CL. The state of women in academic medicine: the pipeline and pathways to leadership, 2013–2014: Association of American Medical Colleges. 2014.
30. Lewiss RE, Silver JK, Bernstein CA, Mills AM, Overholser B, Spector ND. Is academic Medicine making mid-career women physicians invisible? J Womens Health (Larchmt). 2020;29(2):187–92. https://doi.org/10.1089/jwh.2019.7732.
31. McKinsey&Company: McKinsey Global Institute. The power of parity: advancing women's equality in Asia Pacific. April 2018. Retrieved from https://www.mckinsey.com/~/media/McKinsey/Featured%20Insights/Gender%20Equality/The%20power%20of%20parity%20Advancing%20womens%20equality%20in%20Asia%20Pacific/MGI-The-power-of-parity-Advancing-womens-equality-in-Asia-pacific-Executive-summary.pdf.
32. McMurray JE, Linzer M, Konrad TR, Douglas J, Shugerman R, Nelson K. The work lives of women physicians results from the physician work life study. The SGIM career satisfaction study group. J Gen Intern Med. 2000;15(6):372–80.
33. Moss-Racusin CA, Dovidio JF, Brescoll VL, Graham MJ, Handelsman J. Science faculty's subtle gender biases favor male students. Proc Natl Acad Sci U S A. 2012;109(41):16474–9. https://doi.org/10.1073/pnas.1211286109.
34. Narayana S, Roy B, Merriam S, Yecies E, Lee RS, Mitchell JL, Medicine C. Minding the gap: organizational strategies to promote gender equity in academic Medicine during the COVID-19 pandemic. J Gen Intern Med. 2020;35(12):3681–4. https://doi.org/10.1007/s11606-020-06269-0.

35. Noland M, Tyler M. Study: Firms with More Women in the C-Suite Are More Profitable. February 8, 2016. Retrieved from https://hbr.org/2016/02/study-firms-with-more-women-in-the-c-suite-are-more-profitable.
36. Noland M, Moran T, Kotschwar B. Is gender diversity profitable? Evidence from a global survey. 2016. Retrieved from https://EconPapers.repec.org/RePEc:iie:wpaper:wp16-3.
37. Pelley E, Carnes M. When a specialty becomes "Women's work": trends in and implications of specialty gender segregation in Medicine. Acad Med. 2020;95(10):1499–506. https://doi.org/10.1097/acm.0000000000003555.
38. The Physicians Foundation: Struggles, barriers afflict women physicians. Retrieved from https://physiciansfoundation.org/topic/struggles-barriers-afflict-women-physicians/.
39. Sectish TC, Hay WW Jr, Mahan JD, Mendoza FS, Spector ND, Stanton B, Planning C. Blueprint for action: visioning summit on the future of the workforce in Pediatrics. Pediatrics. 2015;136(1):161–9. https://doi.org/10.1542/peds.2014-3493.
40. Shannon G, Jansen M, Williams K, Caceres C, Motta A, Odhiambo A, Mannell J. Gender equality in science, medicine, and global health: where are we at and why does it matter? Lancet. 2019;393(10171):560–9. https://doi.org/10.1016/S0140-6736(18)33135-0.
41. Spector ND, Asante PA, Marcelin JR, Poorman JA, Larson AR, Salles A, Silver JK. Women in Pediatrics: Progress, barriers, and opportunities for equity, diversity, and inclusion. Pediatrics. 2019;144(5) https://doi.org/10.1542/peds.2019-2149.
42. Tsugawa Y, Jena AB, Figueroa JF, Orav EJ, Blumenthal DM, Jha AK. Comparison of hospital mortality and readmission rates for Medicare patients treated by male vs female physicians. JAMA Intern Med. 2017;177(2):206–13. https://doi.org/10.1001/jamainternmed.2016.7875.
43. Women's Wellness Through Equity and Leadership (WEL) Project. Published August 19, 2019. Retrieved from https://drexel.edu/medicine/academics/womens-health-and-leadership/elam/blog/womens-wellness-through-equity-and-leadership-project/

Chapter 5
Women of Color in Pediatrics

Alda Maria Gonzaga and Rita P. Guevara

Introduction

Definitions: The Association of American Medical Colleges (AAMC) defines underrepresented in medicine as those individuals who identify as part of racial and ethnic populations underrepresented in the medical profession compared to the general population. It defines women of color (WOC) as a term used to reflect solidarity among women with multiple layered and intersecting identities who have shared experiences [25]. Intersectionality describes the experiences of individuals living at the intersection of multiple minoritized identities, such as race/ethnicity, gender, sexual orientation, ability, etc. Therefore, all women of color live and work in the intersection of multiple minority identities, i.e., being a woman physician and being a woman of color.

The authors of this chapter acknowledge that there is no one term or word that accurately describes the identities of all groups. The terms "women of color" and "underrepresented in medicine" are used by the AAMC; however, it is important to respectfully inquire and adopt terms used by individuals whenever possible. Examples of other terms include "non-white," "BIPOC" (Black, Indigenous, and People of Color), and "Latinx." The terminology is constantly evolving, and it is important to stay up to date on what is appropriate and ask individuals what terms they prefer.

A. M. Gonzaga
University of Pittsburgh School of Medicine, Pittsburgh, PA, USA
e-mail: gonzagaa@upmc.edu

R. P. Guevara (✉)
Drexel University College of Medicine, Philadelphia, PA, USA
e-mail: rpg34@drexel.edu

N. D. Spector et al. (eds.), *Women in Pediatrics*,
https://doi.org/10.1007/978-3-030-98222-5_5

Brief History

One of the privileges of pediatrics is creating a foundation for child health. With equal intention, reflecting on the contributions women of color have made to the field of pediatrics helps create a foundation for professional health and advancement in current and future pediatricians. Two such historic exemplars are recognized below and are a reminder that diversity in pediatrics has been long standing and impactful.

Dr. Rebecca Lee Crumpler became the first Black woman physician in the United States in 1864 and was the first Black woman physician to publish a book, titled *A Book of Medical Discourses* (Fig. 5.1). This two-volume publication shared Dr. Crumpler's medical advice on maternal and child health, among them the benefits of breastfeeding and the concept of social determinants of health. She wished to make healthcare for women and children accessible, dedicating her book "To mothers, nurses, and all who may desire to mitigate the afflictions of the human race" [17].

Dr. Helen Rodriguez Trias was the first Latina director of the American Public Health Association, as well as a public health expert and a women's rights activist (Fig. 5.2). After graduating medical school from the University of Puerto Rico in 1960, she trained in pediatrics and established the first infant health clinic on the island. She was attuned to how racism in medicine, poverty, and healthcare inequity led to poor health. She founded the Committee to End Sterilization Abuse and served as an advocate for women and children with HIV in New York [13].

Mission, Vision, and Values Guiding Professional Opportunities

As exemplified above, underrepresented women in pediatrics have made and will continue to make powerful, impactful, and innovative contributions to the field. As such, recruitment and retention of underrepresented women in pediatrics is essential to the continued growth and evolution of the field. The demographics of the general population in the United States are constantly changing, and in order to continue to provide culturally effective pediatric care [10], all trainees in pediatrics benefit from training with and learning from physicians of diverse backgrounds. Such educational experiences, whether formal or informal, allow physicians to gain the skills required to practice pediatrics with cultural humility. This is the role of all pediatricians regardless of identity, but those underrepresented in medicine can serve as a bridge to culturally effective care through application of their personal experiences and leadership contributions to education and training. The American Academy of Pediatrics (AAP) recognized in 2013 that enhancing pediatric workforce diversity is an important component of providing culturally effective pediatric care [12].

Between 1993 and 2007, the AAP collected data showing that URM pediatricians self-reported that they were more likely to care for children with public

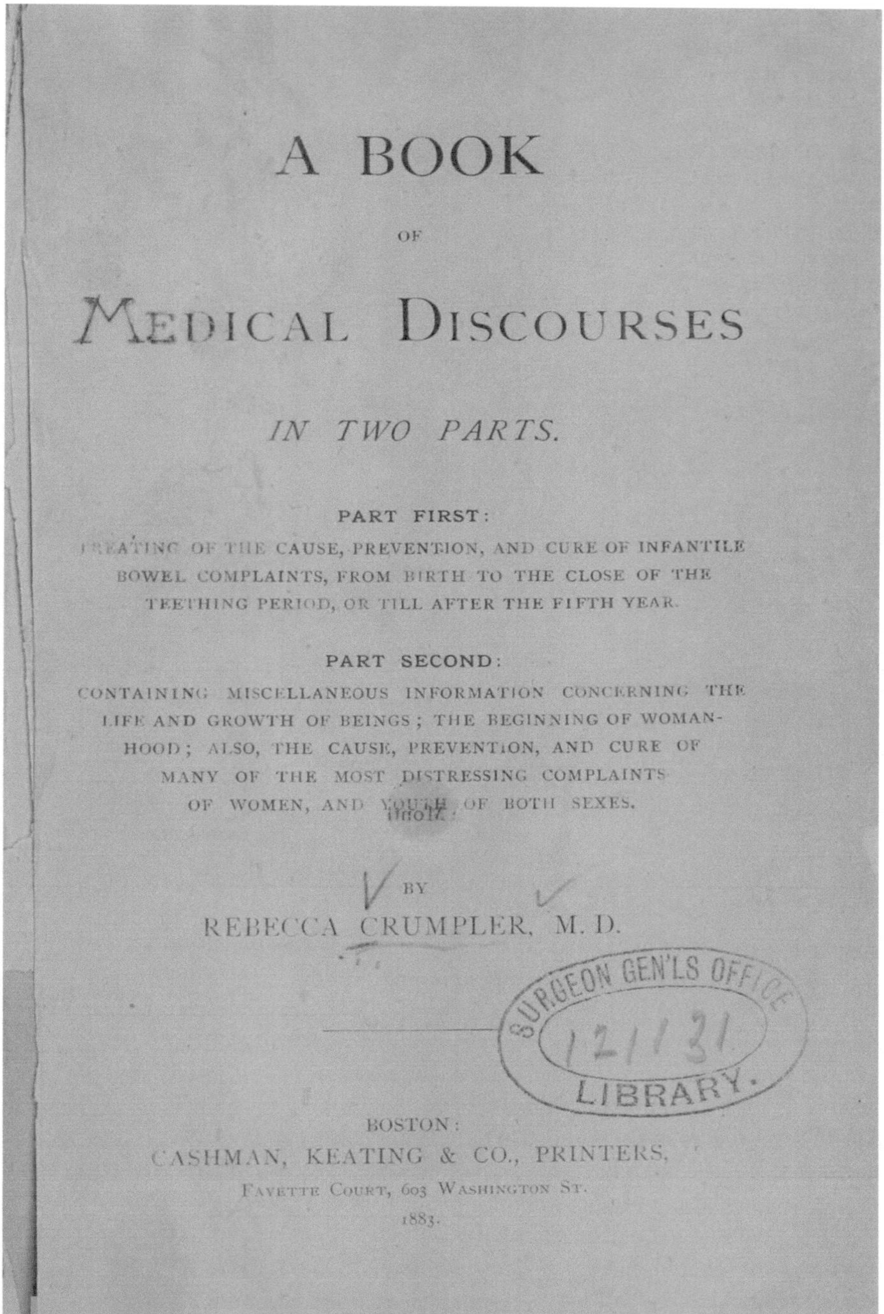

A BOOK

OF

MEDICAL DISCOURSES

IN TWO PARTS.

PART FIRST:

TREATING OF THE CAUSE, PREVENTION, AND CURE OF INFANTILE BOWEL COMPLAINTS, FROM BIRTH TO THE CLOSE OF THE TEETHING PERIOD, OR TILL AFTER THE FIFTH YEAR.

PART SECOND:

CONTAINING MISCELLANEOUS INFORMATION CONCERNING THE LIFE AND GROWTH OF BEINGS; THE BEGINNING OF WOMANHOOD; ALSO, THE CAUSE, PREVENTION, AND CURE OF MANY OF THE MOST DISTRESSING COMPLAINTS OF WOMEN, AND YOUTH OF BOTH SEXES.

BY

REBECCA CRUMPLER, M. D.

BOSTON:

CASHMAN, KEATING & CO., PRINTERS,

FAYETTE COURT, 603 WASHINGTON ST.

1883.

Fig. 5.1 Book cover of *A Book of Medical Discourses: In Two Parts* [1]. There are no known existing photographs of Dr. Crumpler [Crumpler]

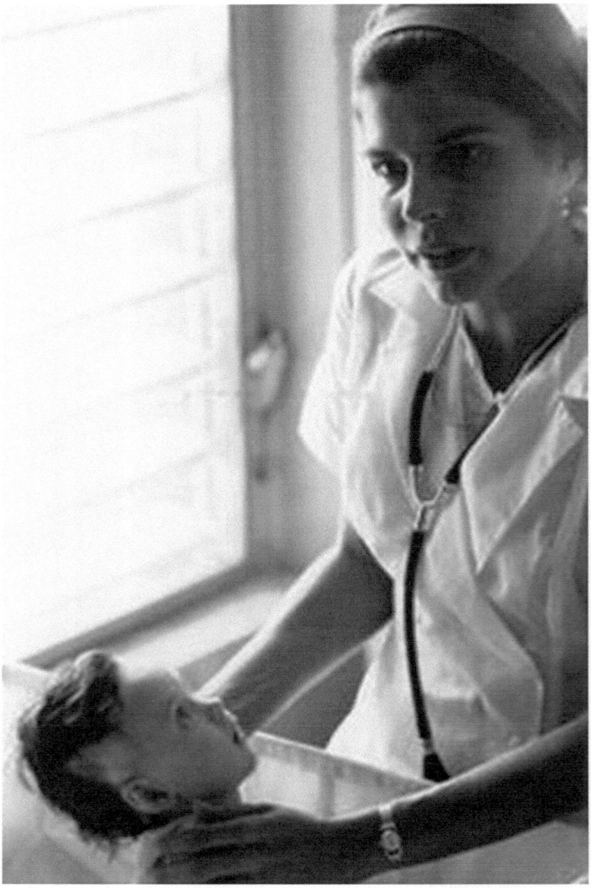

Fig. 5.2 Helen Rodriguez Trias, pediatrician, activist for women's reproductive rights, and founder of the first clinic for newborns on the island of Puerto Rico, ca. 1963. Jim Hansen, photographer, LOOK Magazine Photograph Collection, Library of Congress, Prints & Photographs Division

insurance or no insurance, and who were minorities compared to their non-URM colleagues. This difference was consistent over the duration of the survey period, indicating that URM physicians are caring for a growing population of minority children in this country, many with systemic barriers to healthcare access [9]. A report by the AAMC in 2018 highlighted that when providers have shared life experiences to their patients, including similar demographics, there is an increase in patient satisfaction and adherence to the plan of care [19]. Greenwood et al. in [16] found that racial concordance between Black physicians and Black newborns significantly decreased mortality rates compared to white newborns [16].

There continue to be disparities between the composition of the pediatric workforce and the leadership. Survey data conducted by the AAP in 2019 reported that 14% of respondents identified as Asian, 7% identified as Latino/Hispanic, 4% as Black/African American, and 3% as Other [3]. Looking at AAMC data for women in academic medicine, the largest percentage of URM women faculty were at the instructor and assistant professor levels. Out of all full-time women full professors, only 3% identify as Latina/Hispanic and 2.8% identify as Black/African American, with 1.8% and 1.6% identifying as multiple race non-Hispanic and multiple race Hispanic, respectively [7].

Impact of Non-inclusive Learning and Work Environments

Underrepresented in medicine (URM), as defined at the beginning of this chapter, encompasses a wide scope of identities that can change with changes in the general population. The AAMC definition highlights race and ethnicity, which is the focus of this chapter; however, it can also include other identities such as religion, sexual orientation, gender identity and expression, age, ability, class, and national origin. When an individual is URM, that also implies that their experiences and perspectives may often be missing from the explicit, formal medical curriculum and clinical training. This however *does not* mean that URM individuals are expected to *teach* their colleagues cultural competence or humility. The practice of disproportionately tasking systemic change to a small group of URM individuals is often referred to as the "minority tax," similar to the "woman tax" described by Armijo et al. [6]. This concept was taken a step further by Drs. Ziegelstein and Crews who have coined the term "majority subsidy," defined as "when diversity and inclusion are 'owned' primarily by a small number of persons from underrepresented in medicine (URM) groups and diversity efforts are marginalized…When we farm out diversity in recruitment to a small group, we not only tax them, we also give a subsidy to the people who are not in those groups who should be owning this" [26].

Implicit bias is a positive or negative mental attitude toward a person, thing, or group that a person holds at an unconscious level, which is to say it is outside of their conscious control. While one's implicit biases may be expressed outside of one's awareness and intentionality, its impact is clear to those affected by it. One way implicit biases manifest at an interpersonal level is through microaggressions, whereas those that occur at a structural level are macroaggressions, more commonly called structural or systemic racism/sexism, etc.

As Derald Sue defines them, "Microaggressions are brief and commonplace verbal, behavioral, and environmental indignities, whether intentional or unintentional, that communicate hostile, derogatory, or negative slights and insults that have potentially harmful or unpleasant psychological impact on the target person or group" [23]. Examples of microaggressions include telling someone born and raised in the United States that they speak English really well or endorsing the myth of the meritocracy by stating that everyone can succeed in their country if they work hard enough. Overt discrimination is considered a type of microaggression, subcategorized as microassault. Microassaults tend to be conscious and deliberate expressions of explicit bias (not implicit) that are displayed when an individual loses control or feel safe in engaging in the microassault. Use of racial epithets, the request for a white doctor, and statements endorsing minority inferiority are all examples of microassaults [23].

Intersectionality describes people who live at the intersection of minoritized identities and who often experience a "double jeopardy" of oppressions, in that they may experience microaggressions as a result of any or all of their minoritized identities [22]. Coined by Crenshaw, Eckstrand and colleagues further describe how intersectionality results in interlocking and inseparable cultural patterns of discrimination, and subsequent inequities which cannot be fully understood by only one aspect of identity or experience [14].

Expressions of implicit bias, whether through microaggressions or through biased evaluations, leads to depletion of cognitive bandwidth by those affected. They are faced with the clashing reality that microaggressions are real and "is that what just happened" or did they misinterpret another's actions. This kicks off a reaction which could include doubt, fear, and anger; it can trigger stereotype threat (individuals from minoritized groups perform below their actual abilities fulfilling the negative stereotype associated with their identity group) [11] and disengagement from their work. And as the pervasiveness of microaggressions are invisible to those with power (those of majority identity groups) leads to a lack of acknowledgment of the cumulative effects of frequent microaggressions. In fact, often individuals of majority background do not realize the breadth and depth of discrimination that still exists. Over the long term, the accumulation of biases and microaggressions can lead to negative mental health symptoms, burnout, and for some, leaving the field of medicine entirely [23].

The following table (Table 5.1) outlines some case examples of microaggressions and the impact of the hidden messages within each statement:

Investing in URM Women's Success

Aysola and colleagues have identified six key factors that need to be addressed to foster an inclusive learning and work environment [8]. In addition to acknowledgment of the (1) presence of discrimination and by promoting active bystanders, rather than silent witnesses (2), when microaggressions occur in front of a group of people, other factors were identified.

Addressing the interplay between hierarchy, recognition, and civility (3) by promoting inclusive, equitable organizational policies and procedures that are applied consistently and fairly. URM faculty and learners often feel the rules are applied more stringently to them than to their non-URM peers. Furthermore, ensuring equitable evaluation and promotion standards is key for recognizing URM faculty and learners' accomplishments such that they feel themselves moving upward in the hierarchy of the institution. Likewise, holding all community members, especially those higher in the hierarchy, accountable when they are disrespectful is key to fostering inclusive environment.

Leaders and mentors need to be effective in working with individuals of diverse backgrounds (4). As in the previous domain, leaders and mentors must work to apply expectations consistently and fairly. Sponsoring junior faculty for appropriate

Table 5.1 Example of microaggressions and the hidden messages communicated [23]

Case example	Microaggression theme	Description
A pediatric trainee overhears two advanced practice providers making fun of a child's name in clinic with a similar ethnicity to the trainee	1. *Foreigner in one's own land* – Belief that individuals perceived as racial/ethnic minorities are foreigners 2. *Pathologizing cultural* values [15] – idea that the values and communication styles of people of color are abnormal	1. Here the trainee is witnessing a patient being treated as a foreigner and by association the trainee made to feel like a foreigner as well 2. Here the assumption is that the patient's name does not show assimilation to the dominant culture
Multiple women pediatric trainees of varying heights and appearances who identify as the same race constantly get mistaken for each other	1. *Outgroup homogeneity bias* – Assumptions that members of other groups are similar to each other, in contrast to the diversity of members of one's own group [4] 2. *Second-class citizen* – Treated as less of a person/group compared to the dominant identity/race	1. Because the trainees are viewed as being part of an "other group" (non-white), members of the dominant group (white) view them as the same 2. Members of the dominant group (white) don't take the time to learn the individual identities of the trainees
A Black trainee gets told by one of her attendings that her natural hair is unprofessional	*Pathologizing cultural values*	The attending perceives the trainee's natural hair as not aligning with the dominant (white) culture and therefore unprofessional
A junior faculty URM presents a document she wrote during a meeting with fellow faculty of various ranks, and a white male senior faculty member exclaims with surprise, "wow, you wrote this? It's just so well written!"	*Ascription of intelligence* – Assuming an individual's level of intelligence based on their race/identity	The senior faculty member's comment insinuates that he is surprised by the junior faculty member's intelligence given her race/identity. This could be because she identifies as: URM Junior faculty A woman (or any combination of the above, i.e., intersectionality)

(continued)

Table 5.1 (continued)

Case example	Microaggression theme	Description
A multilingual physician gets interrupted by clinical staff during active patient care to serve as an interpreter for someone else's patient, even though she does not have the training or the time to do so	1. *Foreigner in own land* 2. *Second-class citizen* 3. *Tokenism* – Superficial gesture meant to suggest commitment to a standard [5] 4. *Minority tax* – Placing the burden of systemic change on minority individuals	1. The staff member views the physician as a foreigner who can serve as an interpreter 2. It is assumed that the physician will serve the needs of the staff member in that moment because the staff member's time and needs are more valued than the physician's time/needs 3. Staff member knows they need to use an interpreter, so they choose the physician as a convenient but inappropriate option 4. The physician is given extra work she does not have the training or the protected time to do
A child is admitted to the inpatient service with an unclear diagnosis and her mother, who is phenotypically Black, is labeled by the overnight admitting team as a "poor historian." the day team attending, a bilingual physician, introduces herself and asks the mother for her preferred language. The mother is Spanish-speaking preferred, and the bilingual attending gets a completely different history and physical and determines that the patient's hospital admission was unnecessary	1. *Colorism* – Discrimination against someone with darker skin tone 2. *Outgroup homogeneity bias* 3. *Ascription of intelligence*	1. The night team was quick to assume that the phenotypically Black mother would be a "poor historian" 2. Because the mother appeared Black, she was assumed to be part of a group who are assumed to only speak English 3. This mother was assumed to be less intelligent and therefore a "poor historian" because of her appearance instead of identifying her language preference
A URM physician whose name is often mispronounced is on a committee where multiple white faculty members, junior and senior, often forgo attempting to pronounce people's names, stating "I'm not even going to try"	*Second-class citizen*	The implication with not attempting to pronounce someone's name is that they are less important and are not worth the effort. Since the physician also has experience with their name being mispronounced, they feel less valued by association

leadership positions and/or to participate in high impact scholarship and high impact committees is another key aspect to addressing this factor. Helping URM trainees and faculty connect with role models of similar identity groups fosters the inclusive mindset that it is possible to succeed in the organization as a URM. Many faculty members have found professional coaching to be invaluable to keeping them on track to meet key milestones along their professional trajectory [24].

Supporting the wellness of trainees and faculty (5), especially given the impact of microaggressions and bias on their well-being, is key. This includes creating and promoting affinity groups and safe spaces to discuss recent racially traumatizing events and/or simply the lived experience of working in a space that is dominated by another culture [20]. At UCSF, the decanal staff has formed a Student Rapid Response Team who, within 2 hours of a racial and sociopolitical traumatic event, have sent out an email to students, faculty, and staff acknowledging the event and describing the school's plan for supporting student. Such support includes town halls to discuss the event, mental health resources funded by the school, and delays in exams, among other offerings [21]. Acknowledging the impact of higher levels of indebtedness is an important aspect of well-being to address. Institutions that have loan repayment programs for URM faculty, e.g., those in Maryland who participate in the Maryland State Loan Repayment Program, are able to retain such faculty at their institution for longer periods of time [18]. Furthermore, support for work-life balance (e.g., maternity leave, convenient lactation rooms, etc.) also fosters the sense that URM women faculty are valued within their departments and institutions.

Lastly, creating an environment where there are no perceptions of exclusion to inclusion efforts is important in ensuring a truly inclusive environment (6). Faculty of non-minoritized backgrounds often feel excluded from inclusion efforts, sometimes despite a deep and genuine commitment to this goal. Ensuring all faculty, regardless of background and identity, are invited and included to work on creating an inclusive work environment is key to creating a truly inclusive work and learning environment.

The above factors do not require a mentor or sponsor or ally to have the same overlapping identities as a URM trainee or faculty member. Instead, it is more important for one to have the awareness and understanding of barriers to inclusive learning and work environments. Below is a table (Table 5.2) with specific strategies based on an ally/leader's background.

Conclusion

This chapter provides context to the conversations of diversity, equity, inclusion, and intersectionality for women in pediatrics. If we understand the history of women of color in pediatrics, we will be able to more aptly address the barriers these women face and be able to provide them with effective professional support. This chapter's content serves to plant seeds and cultivate action around awareness and understanding for allies, mentors, and leaders as well as validation, visibility, and support for

Table 5.2 Strategies to be an ally by majority affinity group

Group	Strategies	Examples	Pitfalls to avoid
White colleagues being allies for women of color (WOC)	Do the work of an ally "Walk the walk"	Attend ally group meetings Be an active bystander/upstander Take public action Insist on equitable approaches to hiring and salaries, and promotion and tenure Invite a diverse group of speakers/attendees to the meetings you plan Continue to educate yourself on the experience of WOC and remain curious and open to new terms and identity labels	Don't assume you're an ally; ally is a label you earn Avoid performative allyship Avoid delegating DEI topics or uncomfortable conversations to WOC Don't expect WOC to be the educators on their experience
	Collaborate on advocacy projects – "How can I help?" "what can we do together?"		Don't be paternalistic Check your privilege Avoid being a white savior
	Learn from your WOC colleagues' experiences	Leverage your curiosity and ask women of color to talk about their work, aspirations, and barriers to success Ask WOC to share stories of when someone has been an ally to them	Don't speak on behalf of others
	Work to create conditions where WOC can speak on behalf of themselves and be heard	Ensure WOC are literally sitting at the table	Avoid tokenization (WOC are invited but not given power)
	Spend time getting to know the experience of WOC outside of work	Spend time with WOC outside of work Read articles/books written by WOC in medicine and science (e.g., http://www.gradydoctor.com/) Watch movies/TV programs about WOC in medicine and science	Avoid generalizing the experiences of WOC Don't assume WOC identify with specific racial/ethnic groups; ask if they have a preference for what terms describe them
Women investing in success of women of color	Amplify each other's contributions in meetings	In the Obama administration, women made sure their voices were heard by repeatedly calling attention to their woman colleagues' contributions	Don't speak on behalf of others Don't assume that WOC can only/always speak to DEI topics

Table 5.2 (continued)

Group	Strategies	Examples	Pitfalls to avoid
	Sponsor women of color for leadership roles and awards	e.g., high impact committees Nominate WOC for internal and national (society) leadership roles or awards	Don't be paternalistic Check your privilege Avoid being a white savior
Men investing in the success of women of color	Amplifying their contributions in meetings	"I want to highlight the excellent suggestion XXX just made" White men's voices are still taken more seriously than women or POC voices	Don't speak on behalf of others Avoid referring to WOC as "passionate" or their written/spoken tone as "angry"
	Sponsor women of color for leadership roles and awards	e.g., high impact committees Nominate WOC for internal and national (society) leadership roles or awards	Don't be paternalistic Check your privilege Avoid being a white savior

URM women entering or navigating the field of pediatrics. We highly encourage leaders in pediatrics to collect data and set goals for recruiting and advancing WOC in the field. As Adjo et al. aptly state, "diversity and inclusion without power does not lead us to equity. [2]" Readers are encouraged to reflect on their experiences and how they can utilize the tools and resources shared here to contribute to culturally effective patient care and amplify the work of women pediatricians of color. The field of pediatrics is poised to be a leader in recruiting and supporting WOC succeed and advance in academic medicine.

References

1. A book of medical discourses: in two parts. Crumpler, Rebecca Lee, Boston : Cashman, Keating, printers, 1883 The National Library of Medicine believes this item to be in the public domain https://collections.nlm.nih.gov/catalog/nlm:nlmuid-67521160R-bk.
2. Adjo J, Maybank A, Prakash V. Building inclusive work environments. Pediatrics. 2021;148(supplement 2) Retrieved from https://doi.org/10.1542/peds.2021-051440e.
3. American Academy of Pediatrics, Periodic Survey, 1019 (PS102). 2021. Retrieved from https://downloads.aap.org/AAP/Images/raceeth.png.
4. American Psychological Association definition of outgroup homogeneity bias. (2021). Apa dictionary of psychology. American Psychological Association. Retrieved from https://dictionary.apa.org/outgroup-homogeneity-bias.
5. American Psychological Association definition of tokenism. (2021). Apa dictionary of psychology. American Psychological Association. Retrieved from https://dictionary.apa.org/tokenism.
6. Armijo PR, Silver JK, Larson AR, Asante P, Shillcutt S. Citizenship tasks and women physicians: additional woman tax in academic medicine? J Womens Health (Larchmt). 2020; https://doi.org/10.1089/jwh.2020.8482.
7. Association of American Medical Colleges 2018–2019 The state of women in academic medicine: exploring pathways to equity. Figure 13. Retrieved June 26, 2021., from https://www.aamc.org/data-reports/data/2018-2019-state-women-academic-medicine-exploring-pathways-equity.

8. Aysola J, Barg FK, Martinez AB, Kearney M, Agesa K, Carmona C, Higginbotham E. Perceptions of factors associated with inclusive work and learning environments in health care organizations. JAMA Netw Open. 2018;1(4) https://doi.org/10.1001/jamanetworkopen.2018.1003.
9. Basco WT, Cull WL, O'Connor KG, Shipman SA. Assessing trends in practice demographics of underrepresented minority pediatricians, 1993–2007. Pediatrics. 2010;125(3):460–7. https://doi.org/10.1542/peds.2008-3490.
10. Britton CV, American Academy of Pediatrics Committee on Physician Workforce. Ensuring culturally effective pediatric care: Implications for education and health policy. Pediatrics. 2004;114(6):1677–85. https://doi.org/10.1542/peds.2004-2091.
11. Burgess DJ, Joseph A, van Ryn M, Carnes M. Does stereotype threat affect women in academic medicine? Acad Med. 2012;87(4):506–12. https://doi.org/10.1097/acm.0b013e318248f718.
12. Committee on Pediatric Workforce. Enhancing pediatric workforce diversity and providing culturally effective pediatric care: implications for practice, education, and policy making. Pediatrics. 2013;132(4) https://doi.org/10.1542/peds.2013-2268.
13. "Dr. Helen Rodriguez-Trias." Changing the Face of Medicine. U.S. National Library of Medicine. Last modified June 3, 2015. Retrieved June19, 2021., from https://cfmedicine.nlm.nih.gov/physicians/biography_273.html.
14. Eckstrand KL, Eliason J, St.Cloud T, Potter J. The priority of intersectionality in academic medicine. Acad Med. 2016;91(7):904–7. https://doi.org/10.1097/acm.0000000000001231.
15. Gray A (2019). The bias of "professionalism" standards. Standford social innovation review. Published online June 4, 2019. Retrieved May 11, 2021, from https://ssir.org/articles/entry/the_bias_of_professionalism_standards
16. Greenwood BN, Hardeman RR, Huang L, Sojourner A. Physician–patient racial concordance and disparities in birthing mortality for newborns. Proc Natl Acad Sci. 2020;117(35):21194–200. https://doi.org/10.1073/pnas.1913405117.
17. Klass P. "To mitigate the afflictions of the human race" — the legacy of Dr. Rebecca Crumpler. N Engl J Med. 2021;384(13):1186–9. https://doi.org/10.1056/nejmp2032451.
18. Maryland Higher Education Commission. State Loan Repayment Program (SLRP) and Maryland Loan Assistance Repayment Program for Physicians (MLARP). Retrieved May 11, 2021., from https://mhec.maryland.gov/preparing/Pages/FinancialAid/ProgramDescriptions/prog_mlarp.aspx.
19. Meeks L, Jain N. Accessibility, inclusion, and action in medical education: Lived experiences of learners and physicians with disabilities. 2018. Retrieved June 26, 2021, from https://sds.ucsf.edu/sites/g/files/tkssra2986/f/aamc-ucsf-disability-special-report-accessible.pdf.
20. Personal communication between Alda Maria Gonzaga and Brett Robbins regarding racial healing circles on September 11, 2020.
21. Personal communication between Dr. Gonzaga and Dr. Lee Jones on May 26, 2021.
22. Ruyan AS. What is intersectionality and why is it important? (2018) *Academe*. Nov-Dec 2018. (American Association of University Professors.) Retrieved June 18, 2021, from https://www.aaup.org/article/what-intersectionality-and-why-it-important#.YMzFFuhKiUk.
23. Sue DW, Capodilupo CM, Torino GC, Bucceri JM, Holder AM, Nadal KL, Esquilin M. Racial microaggressions in everyday life: implications for clinical practice. Am Psychol. 2007;62(4):271–86. https://doi.org/10.1037/0003-066x.62.4.271.
24. Williams SN, Thakore BK, McGee R. Coaching to augment mentoring to achieve faculty diversity. Acad Med. 2016;91(8):1128–35. https://doi.org/10.1097/acm.0000000000001026.
25. Underrepresented in medicine definition. AAMC. (2021). Retrieved July 1, 2021, from https://www.aamc.org/what-we-do/equity-diversity-inclusion/underrepresented-in-medicine#:~:text=The%20AAMC%20definition%20of%20underrepresented,numbers%20in%20the%20general%20population.%22.
26. Ziegelstein RC, Crews DC. The majority subsidy. Ann Intern Med. 2019;171(11):845. https://doi.org/10.7326/m19-1923.

Chapter 6
National Campaigns and Organizations Focused on Gender Equity in Pediatrics

Louito Edje, Eliza Lo Chin, and Yemisi Jones

Introduction

Pediatrics is now one of a few fields in medicine dominated by women. One might expect that such a women-predominant field would have a long history of movements and organizations dedicated to achieving equity for women. However, this is not the case. This chapter explores the relatively recent history of organized advocacy and scholarship around disparities for women in pediatrics following a description of efforts within medicine overall. It also explores advocacy around sexually harassing behavior (sexual coercion, unwanted sexual attention, and gender harassment) and the exacerbations of inequity when two or more societal identities intersect in one individual.

History

Despite the high number of women choosing pediatrics as a specialty, leadership in the field has historically been dominated by men. In fact prior to 1971, there were no women in any leadership positions among the major pediatric societies within the Federation of Pediatric Organizations (FOPO) [1]. Prior to 1990, no woman had

L. Edje (✉)
University of Cincinnati Medical Center, Cincinnati, OH, USA
e-mail: edjelc@ucmail.uc.edu

E. L. Chin
American Medical Women's Association, Schaumburg, IL, USA

Y. Jones
Continuing Medical Education, Hospital Medicine, Cincinnati Children's Hospital Medical Center, Cincinnati, OH, USA
e-mail: yemisi.jones@cchmc.org

N. D. Spector et al. (eds.), *Women in Pediatrics*,
https://doi.org/10.1007/978-3-030-98222-5_6

been president of the American Academy of Pediatrics (AAP), the largest of the pediatric associations, and women pediatric department chairs numbered less than ten across the country in any particular year [1]. In 1992, a survey of the salaried physicians in 126 academic departments of pediatrics revealed that fewer women achieved the rank of associate professor or higher, compared to men. The respondents also noted gender disparities in salary, work hours, teaching and patient care responsibilities, mentorship quality, and perceived career barriers [2]. Data from the Association of American Medical Colleges as recently as 2018, show that women comprise only 27.5% of pediatric department chairs, despite representing 58% of full-time women faculty. In addition, the representation of women was more heavily weighted at the rank of instructor (78.4%) compared to full professor (36.5%) [3, 4].

Organizations, Movements, and Campaigns Addressing Gender Equity in Medicine Writ Large

These trends were not specific to pediatrics. Over a 35-year period, women physicians of all specialties in academic medical centers were less likely than men to be promoted to the rank of associate or full professor or to be appointed as department chair, and there was no apparent narrowing in the gap over time [5].

A number of organizations have addressed gender equity in medicine across all specialties including the Association of American Medical Colleges (AAMC); the American Medical Women's Association (AMWA); the American Medical Association Women Physicians Section (AMA-WPS); the *Hedwig van Ameringen* Executive Leadership in Academic Medicine® (ELAM) program; the Center for Women in Academic Medicine and Science (CWAMS); the National Academies of Sciences, Engineering, and Medicine (NASEM); and the Association of Black Women Physicians (ABWP). All have either a mission statement that includes a commitment to gender equity or a statement addressing specific concerns of women physicians or women in academic medicine.

Association of American Medical Colleges

The AAMC has a significant reach with membership including 172 medical schools, over 400 teaching hospitals, over 70 faculty and academic societies, 179,000 full-time faculty, 140,000 residents, and 92,000 medical students. Its mission statement is "Leads and serves the academic medicine community to improve health of people everywhere, dedicated to transforming health through medical education, health care, medical research, and community collaborations" [6]. The AAMC Statement on Gender Equity acknowledges that "equity is a key factor in achieving excellence in academic medicine" [7]. In addition, the AAMC has a subgroup, the Group on

Women in Medicine and Science (GWIMS), which serves both as a network of support and a community focused on advancing women physicians in academia across all specialties [8]. There are institutional affiliations of this larger group which help foster mentorship and sponsorship relationships for early career and mid-career women. Within this group, there is connective tissue between members which includes a newsletter, faculty development seminars, and opportunities to present scholarly work. The AAMC is also committed, along with its member institutions, to intentional identification of practices which exclude women. One example of a resource which elevates the awareness of gender equity is the annual *State of Women in Academic Medicine* report which presents a snapshot of the representation of women at key points along the academic medicine pipeline. This report can be used to "turn data into action to advance women at your institution" [9].

American Medical Women's Association

AMWA, founded in 1915, is the oldest multispecialty organization to advance women in medicine. Its membership includes not only physicians, residents, and medical students but also the pipeline of premedical students, other disciplines in the health professions, and supporters. Its mission is to advance women in medicine, advocate for equity, and ensure excellence in healthcare [10].

AMWA has a Gender Equity Taskforce whose mission is to "strive to accomplish gender equity as a fact of life in society, and to engage in activities, actions, and collaborations pursuant to this goal, beginning with the healthcare industry, of which women physicians are one component." The goals of the organization are to raise awareness of, and advocate for, the importance of gender equity; form supportive networks, including a speakers bureau; provide opportunities to recognize and elevate the work of women physicians; as well as provide funds and other resources such as the Linda Brodsky Grant which supports work that promotes gender equity, medical student success, clinical research, and the advancement of women physicians [11]. Revolution by Resolution: Advancing Gender Equity in Medical Societies, State by State is an effort to promote gender equity resolutions within each state medical society, modeled after resolutions passed within the American Medical Association (AMA) and the Massachusetts Medical Society [11]. The work of AMWA addresses issues faced by women physicians at every stage of their career from premedical student to retired physician.

American Medical Association

In 1979, the AMA founded the ad hoc Committee on Women Physicians to encourage the membership and participation of women physicians throughout organized medicine. In 1997, the AMA created the Women Physicians Congress (WPC) as an advocacy and networking forum dedicated to women in medicine. In 2013, the AMA established the Women Physicians Section (WPS) which currently represents more than 100,000 women physicians and medical students. Its opt-out model encompasses all AMA members who identify as women [12, 13]. While the AMA WPS focuses its policy compendium on issues that affect women, the Section is open to all physicians within the AMA. This encourages allyship. It also collaborates with other organizations for the benefit of mutual goals via networking, mentoring, and leadership development. The WPS also monitors trends that affect all women across medicine, providing a policy platform to amplify member concerns.

Executive Leadership in Academic Medicine®

ELAM®, established in 1995, is a 1-year fellowship for qualified women who have achieved the rank of associate professor or higher. This admission criterion for application is consistent with the fact that women associate and full professors are 50% less likely than their counterparts to be appointed as department chair. This leadership fellowship provides coaching, networking, and mentoring across the health professions. The goal is to maximize the leadership potential of women for executive leadership positions in academia [14].

CWAMS was founded in 2019 to address the persistent challenges of gender inequity which have limited progress for women in medicine and to "connect women to the resources, networks, and information they need" to advance their careers. Its programs include a national Faculty Network and a group for women in senior leadership positions, known as the Organization of Women Leaders (OWL) [15].

National Academies of Sciences, Engineering, and Medicine

The National Academies of Sciences, Engineering, and Medicine (NASEM) is a nonprofit organization comprised of three honorific societies (the National Academy of Sciences, National Academy of Engineering, and National Academy of Medicine) whose members are elected based on academic achievements. Its mission is to "advise the nation and provide independent, objective advice to inform policy with evidence, spark progress and innovation, and confront challenging issues for the benefit of society" [16]. While the historic archive of its member organization – the National Academy of Sciences – had men as president from 1863 through 2016, the NASEM has been intentional in its progress toward equity as evidenced by its 2018 Report to Congress. This included a study that examined the effects of sexually harassing behavior on the career paths of women in its member professions [17].

The National Academy of Medicine, founded in 1970 as the Institute of Medicine (IOM), operated under the 1863 Congressional Charter of the NAS with the mission to improve health for all by advancing science, accelerating health equity, and providing independent, authoritative, and trusted advice nationally and globally. It is one of the highest honors in medicine to be elected to this elite body of just over 2000 members. In 2019, 40% of new members were women [18]. In 2014, 11.4% of the newly 70 newly elected members were Black, with six of eight being women [19].

Association of Black Women Physicians

ABWP is a nonprofit organization committed to "the improvement of public health and welfare, through the advancement of knowledge concerning women and the community health." This organization, established in 1982 by 50 women discussing career development, funds projects that address the health and wellness of underserved communities and are committed to improving the quality of life of future and current Black women physicians [20].

In addition to these large national organizations, other programs like the Women in Medicine Summit (WIMS); GRIT for Women in Medicine: Growth, Resilience, Inspiration, and Tenacity, Brave Enough; and Promoting and Respecting Our Women Doctors (PROWD) have provided training, education, and/or communities of support to empower women physicians [21–24]. In addition, there have been broader efforts that have included other health professions, for example, TIME's UP Healthcare [25].

Gender Equity and Sexual Harassment Awareness Campaigns

Women in medicine are using social media more than they were in the past. 18.5% are active users, which is 21% up from the previous year of 2015.

Physician Moms Group (PMG) is an international online community of over 115,000 physician mothers founded in 2014 to share advice on parenting as physicians [26].

500 Women in Medicine, a part of 500 Women Scientists, comprised of over 20,000 women from over 100 countries, was started in 2016 by four graduate students who determined to be committed to speaking up for science and marginalized populations in science [27]. GirlMedMedia, and other online communities for women in medicine, developed with a social focus but has been a forum for sharing experiences related to gender inequity.

The advent of social media as an avenue to amplify messages about gender inequity brought with it several inexpensive, highly visible campaigns that shed light on sex-based harassment in medicine and defied the stereotype of what a physician looks like. One such Twitter ™ hashtag, #IlookLikeASurgeon, was launched in August 2015, when two surgical residents at the University of North Carolina at Chapel Hill were inspired by #ILookLikeAnEngineer, a campaign of women engineers posting pictures of themselves on social media in T-shirts with the hashtag. This campaign subsequently was picked up by the Association of Women Surgeons. Women surgeons tweeted pictures of their authentic selves. One depicts Johns Hopkins trauma surgeon, Dr. Catherine Velopulos, in her high heels in the operating room, defying the white trifecta (white coat, white skin, white hair) [28]. This movement largely showed the authentic side of women surgeons from the operating room setting to life outside medicine at home with colleagues and children [29]. #ILookLikeASurgeon had generated more than 128 million impressions by September 2015, nearly 40,000 individual tweets, and more than 7900 participants, and those numbers continue to grow [30]. In 2017, the movement resurfaced in NY magazine [30].

Dr. Julie Silver, Associate Professor and Associate Chair in the Department of Physical Medicine and Rehabilitation at Harvard Medical School, leads the Harvard Career Advancement and Leadership Skills for Women in Healthcare. In recent years, she has launched annual strategic initiatives with associated campaign hashtags to target workforce gender disparities: #QuoteHer (2016) to elevate women physician voices in publishing; Walls Do Talk Challenge (2017) to counter gender stereotypes in medical education; #BeEthical (2018) to "recognize that workforce gender equity is an ethical imperative"; #NeedHerScience (2019) to "address journal-level gender bias"; #HerTimeIsNow (2020) to address gender inequities and equitability of women in their spheres of influence; and #GiveHerAReasonToStay in healthcare (2021) to help stem the efflux of women from healthcare. These campaigns have focused on some, or all, of the "gatekeepers of academic medicine," namely, medical schools, hospitals, and healthcare institutions, medical journals, medical societies, and funding sources. They have been instrumental in using data to drive change and pointing out that there are enough qualified women to fill top leadership positions [31–36].

Intersectionality

Intersectionality, a legal term first coined in 1989 by civil rights advocate, philosopher, and Professor of Law at UCLA, Kimberly Crenshaw, is the intersection of two or more social identities. These often exacerbate the inequities experienced in a single identity [37].

We know women are paid less than men. Put another way, on average, women have to work until the beginning of April to make the same salary as male counterparts made the previous year [38]. But Black women are paid even less than white women (Fig. 6.1).

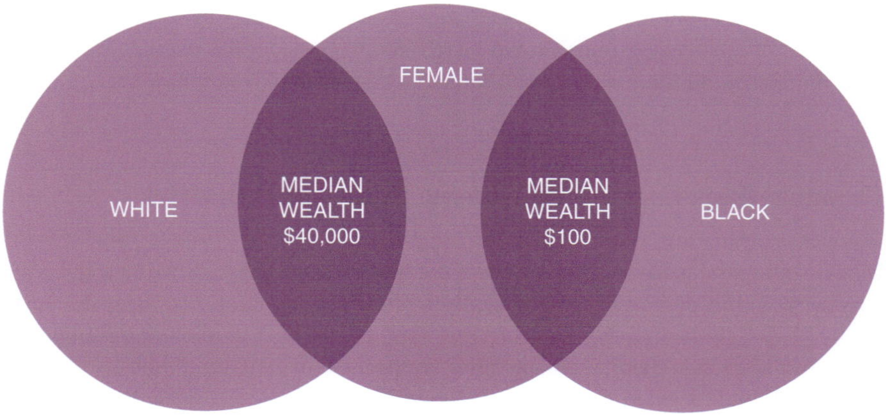

Fig. 6.1 Intersectionality of gender and race exacerbates pay and wealth inequities [37]

The effects of intersectionality are also evident when you consider the number of women physicians who become department chairs is 18%, while the percentage of Black women department chairs is 12% of that 18% [39].

There are organizations which have had a positive impact in intersectionality with their choice of leadership. By way of example, the American College of Surgeons just hired an executive director who is the first Black women surgeon to hold this role [40]. Another is the Society of Black Academic Surgeons which amplifies the voices of Black women by collaborating with other organizations such as the Association of Women Surgeons, Michigan, and the Michigan Women's Surgical Collaborative [41].

A third example of intersectionality's effects is the impact that the COVID-19 pandemic had on women overall, and Black women physicians in particular. Before the pandemic, women reported increased domestic and childcare obligations which averaged 8.5 hours more per week as compared to men [42].

This disproportionate amount of time was further compounded by the need to balance such activities as managing homeschooling when schools had closed for safety. Black women, who make up only 2.6% of all physicians [43], had the compounded stress brought on by issues of racism in the wake of George Floyd's death and the burden of needing to advocate for Black and Brown communities which have not only been affected by higher death rates and hospitalization due to COVID-19 but also by decreased access to vaccines [44]. This additional work is often done in their spare time outside of work, thus decreasing opportunities for other scholarly activity.

Spector and Overholser pointed out that during the pandemic, the number of first authors decreased by 19% as compared to the same time the previous year [45]. It is likely that this decrease will have downstream effects with promotions to higher academic ranks. One survey, for example, found that 10% more women medical students worry about the effects of COVID-19 on their careers as compared to men [46]. Foci of advocacy groups should be tailored to consider the intersectionality of their members and the variable need for support within a given initiative.

Organizations Focused on Gender Equity in Pediatrics

Despite being the medical specialty with the highest percentage of women (64.3%), advocacy within pediatrics only recently started gaining momentum in the early 2000s [47]. Scholarship highlighting the issue began with studies describing disparities in academic medicine and started to increase in 2010s with the publication of the first studies examining gender inequity in academic pediatric departments. Rotbart et al. described differences at a single institution in male and female faculty attainment of senior academic rank, leadership positions, as well as pay gap [48]. There were subsequent publications including a call to action to end gender inequity in academic medicine [49]; descriptions of disparities in reviewer pool, invited editorials, and editorial boards [49, 50]; and demonstration of pay and leadership gaps within pediatrics [51–54]. Other publications during this period highlighted the differences in household responsibilities between men and women pediatricians [55]. The publication of Spector et al.'s framework for a comprehensive, stepwise approach to achieve gender equity occurred in *Pediatrics*, in 2019 [56].

Formalized advocacy mirrored the increased awareness in the literature evidenced by the creation of the first FOPO task force on Women in Pediatrics in 2006. This report identified the need for more women physician leaders and highlighted key issues relevant to women, such as part-time work options, flexible career paths for physician-scientists, and availability of high-quality childcare [1]. A second task force was convened in 2007 to further this work [57]. Since that time, various initiatives and groups dedicated to supporting women in pediatrics have evolved in each of the member organizations.

Academic Pediatric Association

The Academic Pediatric Association (APA) has a Women in Medicine special interest group which has as its aim to "address the issues facing women in academic pediatrics" [58]. Its focus is on areas of disparities including salaries, academic advancement, negotiating skills, integrating professional, and personal lives, confronting sexual harassment and intimidation, part-time employment, and leadership opportunities. Much of the output of the group is focused on educating and supporting its members.

American Academy of Pediatrics

The American Academy of Pediatrics (AAP) is one of the co-sponsors of the Women's Wellness through Equity and Leadership (WEL) project along with American Academy of Family Physicians, American College of Obstetricians and Gynecologists, American College of Physicians, American Psychiatric Association, and American Hospital Association [59]. This project aims to improve gender disparities for women physicians by bringing together a small cohort of early and mid-career women from across the different organizations to participate in workshops, meetings, and focused mentoring [60]. The AAP also has a Committee on Pediatric Workforce (COPW) which studies the impact of gender on the pediatric workforce and makes corresponding recommendations [61]. This committee has served as a forum for women pediatricians to share their insights on relevant topics over the years. Several subspecialty sections within the AAP have committees targeting women physicians, including Women in Neonatology [60] and Women in Pediatric Hospital Medicine [62]. These groups work to support the women in their field with career and professional development as well as provide advocacy and networking opportunities.

American Pediatric Society

The American Pediatric Society (APS) partners with and supports various initiatives aimed at workforce diversity such as the Pediatric Scientist Development Program which aims to increase and diversify the pediatric scientist workforce through an intensive training program [63]. Journeys and Frontiers in Pediatric Research is another program that supports pediatric researchers and focuses on inclusion of members from groups traditionally underrepresented in medicine [64]. The APS Committee on Diversity, Inclusion & Equity was established in 2012 and helps guide these efforts and others for the Society [63].

In addition to the work within established pediatric organizations, various movements and independent groups have also launched to support women in pediatrics. ADVANCE PHM was founded to accelerate gender equity in pediatric hospital medicine and has initiatives focused on education, advocacy, research, career development, and cultivating allies [64]. Women in Pediatrics is focused on developing leadership and entrepreneurial skills in women pediatricians through online networking and in-person retreats [65]. Many pediatricians have also been active in the social media-focused movements mentioned above as well as parts of closed communities on platforms such as Facebook.

Gender Equity in Other Organizations with a Predominance of Women Physicians

Second to pediatrics in numbers of women physicians is obstetrics and gynecology, notably the first surgical specialty to have a majority of members who are women. In the AAMC 2020 Physician Specialty Report, women comprised 58.9% of the physician workforce within the field [47]. Within this specialty, however, the literature on organized advocacy for women in medicine has also been more recent. A review in 2020 by Heisler et al. is found persistent gender-related biases, discrimination, and sexual harassment, as well as a gender wage gap, despite correcting for other variables [66]. In fact, the "critical mass" in numbers has not translated into more equitable opportunities for women within the field. Worse yet, the predominance of women in the field has resulted in what some would characterize as a feminization of the specialty, with gynecologic surgery being viewed as "women's work," leading to a decline in salaries and status for those physicians [67].

In 2018, Baecher-Lind et al. issued a call to action, in response to an incident at the national meeting where a prominent leader displayed a highly inappropriate photo [68, 69]. The authors of this paper note that this incident and the ensuing response pointed to a pervasive culture of gender inequity and sexual harassment enabled by what was felt to be a relative silence among specialty leaders regarding these injustices – despite recent attention within medicine for the #MeToo movement and other advocacy campaigns [69]. The following year, the American College of Obstetricians and Gynecologists established a Diversity, Equity, and Inclusive Excellence (DEIE) Workgroup to ensure a diverse, equitable, and inclusive workforce within the field [70].

Women in Medicine Organizations

Why was the formal organization of women physicians much later within fields like pediatrics and obstetrics and gynecology? Could it be that higher numbers of women physicians decreased the impetus for the formal networking groups and the need for a separate association or section? Or did the increased numbers convey a passive reassurance that masked the reality of underlying gender inequities? Within these specialties, the pipeline of women no longer seems to be the issue in terms of absolute numbers, yet research continues to document gender disparities in pay, academic promotion, bias, and harassment and underrepresentation of certain groups [66]. The lived experience of women physicians within these specialties reinforces the hypothesis that change will result not from a "critical mass" of individuals but from the presence of "critical actors" who will drive change [66, 71].

In looking across the wider landscape of medicine, particularly in fields with fewer women, we see an earlier rise of women in medicine specialty groups. It might be hypothesized that the need for establishing a network of support may have been greater in these specialties where women were underrepresented, both to foster professional networking and provide a united platform for promoting change. One of the earliest groups was the Women's Dermatologic Society, founded in 1973 [72]. Others soon followed, and the 1980s saw a rise of additional groups, including the Society of Women in Urology (1980), Association of Women Surgeons and American Association for Women in Radiology (1981), the Association of Women Psychiatrists, Ruth Jackson Orthopaedic Society, and Women in Nephrology (1983), the American Association of Women Emergency Physicians (1985), Women in Thoracic Surgery (1986), and Women in Neurosurgery and Women in Ophthalmology (1989) [73–82]. Table 6.1 lists various women in medicine specialty groups or sections that are currently in existence today.

Alliances that bring together these various groups will help amplify the voice of women physician leaders. WEL 2.0 led by AAP has expanded to include an additional four organizations, the American Medical Association (AMA), American Medical Women's Association (AMWA), National Hispanic Medical Association (NHMA), and National Medical Association (NMA) [83]. AMWA launched a Networking Alliance in 2010 to convene various associations around the common goals of advancing women physicians [84]. The nascent formation of a Gender Equity in Academic Medicine and Science (GEMS) Alliance [9] may serve to bring organizational groups together, strengthening the voice of women in medicine and forging collaborations among "critical actors" across specialties to be a unified voice.

Conclusion

The past few decades have seen tremendous growth in the number of organizations supporting women in medicine, both across and within specialties as well as within institutions. These groups provide avenues of change within the profession through organized efforts and collective advocacy. By raising awareness of issues surrounding gender equity, workplace discrimination, implicit and explicit biases, and more, they have worked through traditional advocacy channels as well as harnessed the power of social media and digital technology to amplify their messages to a much wider audience. Some groups, like AMWA, AMA-WPS, CWAMS, and PMG, are multidisciplinary, promoting collaboration across specialties. Others work within specialties to advocate for change. Joining forces around a common goal may be an effective way to promote change as organizations collaborate with each other and forge alliances.

Despite the rise of numbers of women in medicine, the gender gap in leadership still persists. The relatively stagnant numbers of women in top leadership positions indicates that much work is yet to be done. While women are now a majority of entering medical students, we need to invest in programs that promote women's leadership, because ultimately, change may result not from overall numbers but

Table 6.1 Women in medicine organizations

General women in medicine organizations	Year founded	Website	Reference (note, these are references for column B, the year of founding)
American Medical Association (AMA) Women Physicians Section (WPS)	2013	https://www.ama-assn.org/member-groups-sections/women-physicians	[13]
American Medical Women's Association (AMWA)	1915	amwa-doc.org	[8]
Association of American Medical Colleges Group on Women in Medicine and Science (GWIMS)	2009	https://www.aamc.org/professional-development/affinity-groups/gwims	[85]
Center for Women in Academic Medicine and Science (CWAMS)	2019	https://cwams.org/	[86]
Hedwig van Ameringen Executive Leadership in Academic Medicine® (ELAM)	1995	https://drexel.edu/medicine/academics/womens-health-and-leadership/elam/about-elam/	[87]
National Osteopathic Women Physicians Associatiion (NOWPA)	1904		[88]
WOMEN in Medicine Specialty Organizations			
Academic Pediatric Association Women in Medicine SIG		academicpeds.org/sig/women-in-medicine	
Academy for Women in Academic Emergency Medicine (AWAEM)	2009	https://www.saem.org/about-saem/academies-interest-groups-affiliates2/awaem	[89]
Advance PHM	2021	https://www.advancephm.org/	[90]
American Academy of Pediatrics (AAP) Section on Hospital Medicine (SOHM) Women in Pediatric Hospital Medicine (PHM) Subcommittee	2020	www.sohmlibrary.org/women-in-phm.html	[91]
American Association for Women in Radiology (AAWR)	1981	https://www.aawr.org	[75]

Table 6.1 (continued)

General women in medicine organizations	Year founded	Website	Reference (note, these are references for column B, the year of founding)
American Association of Women Emergency Physicians (AAWEP)	1985	https://www.acep.org/how-we-serve/sections/american-association-of-women-eps/welcome-to-american-association-of-women-emergency-physicians/#sm.000qn3krlrdte1j11qh1dt64e53jl	[79]
American Pediatric Association Women in Pediatrics Women in Pediatrics Interest Group		https://www.academicpeds.org/sig/women-in-medicine	
Association of Women in Rheumatology (AWIR)	2015	http://www.awirgroup.org	[92]
Association of Women Psychiatrists (AWP)	1983	http://associationofwomenpsychiatrists.com/executive-committee/	[76]
Association of Women Surgeons (AWS)	1981	https://www.womensurgeons.org	[74]
FeminEM	2015	https://feminem.org/	[93]
Ruth Jackson Orthopedic Society (RJOS)	1983	http://rjos.org/	[77]
Society for Women in Radiation Oncology (SWRO)	2017	https://www.societywomenradiationoncology.com/	[94]
Society of Cardiothoracic Anesthesiologists (SCA) Women in Cariodthoracic Anesthesiologist (WICTA)	2018	http://www.thoracic-anesthesia.com/?page_id=5	[95]
Society of Women in Urology (SWIU)	1980	www.swiu.org	[73]
Women in Anesthesiology (WIA)	2014	https://www.womeninanesthesiology.org/	[96]
Women in Cardiology Section (WIC) American College of Cardiology (ACC)	2005	https://www.acc.org/membership/sections-and-councils/women-in-cardiology-section	[97]
Women in Emergency Medicine Section (WiEMS) American Academy of Emergency Medicine (AAEM)	2020	https://www.aaem.org/get-involved/sections/wiems	[98]

(continued)

Table 6.1 (continued)

General women in medicine organizations	Year founded	Website	Reference (note, these are references for column B, the year of founding)
Women in Endocrinology (WIE)	1977-1978	https://www.women-in-endo.org/	[99]
Women in Endoscopy (WIE)	2016	http://www.womeninendo.org/leaders	[100]
Women in Nephrology (WIN)	1983	http://www.womeninnephrology.org/	[78]
Women in Neurosurgery (WINS)	1989	www.neurosurgerywins.org	[81]
Women in Ophthalmology (WIO)	1989	https://www.wioonline.org	[82]
Women in Otolaryngology (WIO) Section of the American Academy of Otolaryngology - Head and Neck Surgery	2010	https://www.entnet.org/get-involved/sections/women-in-otolaryngology/	[101]
Women in Pediatrics	2019	womeninpeds.com	[102]
Women in Rhinology (WiR) Section of the American Rhinologic Society (ARS)	2019	https://www.american-rhinologic.org/women-in-rhinology-section	[103]
Women in Surgery Committee, American College of Surgeons		https://www.facs.org/about-acs/governance/acs-committees/women-in-surgery-committee	
Women in Thoracic Surgery (WTS)	1986	https://wtsnet.org/	[80]
Women's Dermatologic Society (WDS)	1973	https://www.womensderm.org/	[72]
Women's Neurologists Group (WNG)	2015	https://twitter.com/wngtweets?lang=en	[104]
Other women in medicine organizations			
Women in Medicine (WIM)	1984	https://womeninmedicine.org	[105]
Jewish Orthodox Women's Medical Association (JOWMA)	2019	https://www.jowma.org/	[106]
Association of Black Women Physicians (ABWP)	1982	https://www.blackwomenphysicians.org/	[107]

from the work of "critical actors." We also need to recognize that even as the numbers of overall women increase, efforts are still needed to ensure equal representation of diverse groups and recognition of intersectionality and the compounding of multiple inequities beyond gender. Given the predominance of women in pediatrics and the growing advocacy efforts within the field, this specialty is perfectly positioned to lead the way to a future where all women in medicine can realize their full potential.

References

1. Stanton B, et al. A change in the pediatric leadership landscape. J Pediatr. 2011;158(3):347–348 e2. https://www.ncbi.nlm.nih.gov/pubmed/21316523. Accessed online: 6.28.21.
2. Kaplan SH, et al. Sex differences in academic advancement — results of a National Study of Pediatricians. N Engl J Med. 1996;335(17):1282–90. https://www.nejm.org/doi/full/10.1056/NEJM199610243351706. Accessed online: 6.28.21.
3. Association of American Medical Colleges. 2018–2019 The state of women in academic medicine: exploring pathways to equity.. https://www.aamc.org/data-reports/data/2018-2019-state-women-academic-medicine-exploring-pathways-equity. Accessed online 11.6.21.
4. Association of American Medical Colleges. 2018 U.S. medical school faculty.. https://www.aamc.org/data-reports/faculty-institutions/interactive-data/data-reports/faculty-institutions/interactive-data/2018-us-medical-school-faculty. Accessed online 11.6.21.
5. Richter KP, et al. Women physicians and promotion in academic medicine. N Engl J Med. 2020;383(22):2148–57. https://www.nejm.org/doi/full/10.1056/NEJMsa1916935. Accessed online: 6.28.21.
6. Association of American Medical Colleges: Who We Are. https://www.aamc.org/who-we-are. Accessed Online: Accessed online: 6.28.21.
7. AAMC Statement on Gender Equity. https://www.aamc.org/what-we-do/equity-diversity-inclusion/aamc-statement-gender-equity. Accessed Online: Accessed online: 6.28.21.
8. AAMC Group on Women in Medicine and Science (GWIMS). https://www.aamc.org/professional-development/affinity-groups/gwims. Accessed Online: 6.28.21.
9. 2013–2014 The State of Women in Academic Medicine: The Pipeline and Pathways to Leadership. https://www.aamc.org/data-reports/data/2013-2014-state-women-academic-medicine-pipeline-and-pathways-leadership. Accessed online: 6.28.21.
10. About AMWA. https://www.amwa-doc.org/about-amwa/.
11. AMWA Gender Equity Task Force. https://www.amwa-doc.org/our-work/initiatives/gender-equity-task-force/.
12. AMA Women Physicians Section (WPS). https://www.ama-assn.org/member-groups-sections/women-physicians.
13. A Profile & History of Women in Medicine. American Medical Association. https://cdn.ymaws.com/msdc.site-ym.com/resource/resmgr/eNewsline/2016-history-women-in-medici.pdf. Accessed online 11.6.21.
14. The Hedwig van Ameringen Executive Leadership in Academic Medicine® (ELAM). https://drexel.edu/medicine/academics/womens-health-and-leadership/elam/. Accessed online 6.15.21.
15. When women lead, cultures change. CWAMS. https://cwams.org/who-we-are/. Accessed online 6.15.21.
16. Who We Are: Created to Advise the Nation. The National Academies of Sciences Engineering, Medicine. https://www.nationalacademies.org/about. Accessed online 6.15.21.
17. Sexual Harassment in Academic Science, Engineering, and Medicine. https://www.nationalacademies.org/our-work/sexual-harassment-in-academia, . Accessed online: 6.28.21.

18. Women nearly 40 percent of new members of National Academy of medicine. WIA Report, 2019. https://www.wiareport.com/2019/01/women-make-up-nearly-40-percent-of-the-new-members-of-the-national-academy-of-medicine/. Accessed online 9.19.21.
19. Eight African Americans elected to the National Academy of medicine. The Journal of Blacks in Higher Education, 2019. https://www.jbhe.com/2017/01/eight-african-americans-elected-to-the-national-academy-of-medicine/. Accessed online 9.19.21.
20. Committed to Improved Public Health and Welfare. https://www.blackwomenphysicians.org/about-us.
21. An evolution of empowerment. Women in Medicine. https://www.womeninmedicinesummit.org/.
22. Harris CE, et al. GRIT: women in medicine leadership conference participants' perceptions of gender discrimination, disparity, and mitigation. Mayo Clinic Proceedings April 30, 2021. https://www.mcpiqojournal.org/article/S2542454821000400/abstract.
23. Brave Enough: Teaching Women Work-Life Control. https://www.becomebraveenough.com/.
24. Promoting and Respecting Our Women Doctors (PROWD), twitter.com/prowdwomen?lang=en. Accessed 11.6.21..
25. TIME'S UP Healthcare: We're here to heal a broken system. timesupfoundation.org/work/times-up-healthcare. Accessed 11.6.21.
26. Physician Moms Group (PMG). https://mypmg.com/About. Accessed online: 5.28.21.
27. 500 Women in Medicine. https://500womenscientists.org/updates/2018/12/2/500-women-in-medicine. Accessed online: 5.28.21.
28. Vartabedian B. What does a surgeon look like? – a defining hashtag. 33 Charts. https://33charts.com/surgeon-look-like. Accessed online 11.6.21.
29. #ILookLikeASurgeon goes viral: How it happened. https://bulletin.facs.org/2015/11/ilooklikeasurgeon-goes-viral-how-it-happened. Accessed online: 5.28.21.
30. #ILookLikeASurgeon healthcare social media hashtag. www.symplur.com/healthcare-hashtags/ilooklikeasurgeon/. Accessed online: 5.28.21.
31. Silver J. Invisible women: Female doctors and health care leaders are being hidden in plain sight. Stat News. October 24, 2016. https://www.statnews.com/2016/10/24/female-doctors-invisible-women/. Accessed 11.6.21.
32. PR Underground. Doctor launches 'walls do talk' challenge to combat gender stereotypes in medical schools. October 20, 2017. https://www.prunderground.com/doctor-launches-walls-do-talk-challenge-to-combat-gender-stereotypes-in-medical-schools/00107381/. Accessed 11.6.21.
33. A Call to Healthcare Leaders: Ending Gender Workforce Disparities is an Ethical Imperative (v4). September 17, 2018 https://sheleadshealthcare.com/wp-content/uploads/2018/09/Be-Ethical-Campaign.pdf. Accessed online: 11.6.21.
34. Silver JK. Tips for Publishing in Journals. September 26, 2019. http://sheleadshealthcare.com/wp-content/uploads/2019/09/NHS_Infographic.pdf Accessed online: 5.28.21.
35. Silver J. Her Time Is Now Report (v2). September 1, 2020. https://sheleadshealthcare.com/wp-content/uploads/2020/09/HerTimeIsNow_Report.pdf. Accessed 11.6.21.
36. Silver J. Give Her A Reason to stay in healthcare (v1). August 1, 2021. https://sheleadshealthcare.com/wp-content/uploads/2021/07/GiveHerAReasonToStay-Infographic.pdf . Accessed 11.6.21.
37. Steinmetz K. She coined the term 'intersectionality' over 30 years ago. Here's what it means to Her today. February 20, 2020. https://time.com/5786710/kimberle-crenshaw-intersectionality/?amp=true. Accessed online 7.5.21.
38. Here's How Much Longer Women Have to Work to Earn the Same as Men. Care.com. February 26, 2018. https://www.care.com/c/equal-pay-day-gender-pay-gap-by-profession. Accessed online: 6.28.21.
39. Paturel A. Where are all the Women Deans. AAMC. https://www.aamc.org/news-insights/where-are-all-women-deans. Accessed online: 6.28.21.

40. The Next ACS Executive Director. American College of Surgeons Bulletin Brief. https://www.facs.org/publications/bulletin-brief/060821/executive-director. Accessed online: 6.28.21.
41. Society of Black Academic Surgeons Annual Meeting. September 7,2018. https://medicine.umich.edu/dept/surgery/news/archive/201809/society-black-academic-surgeons-annual-meeting. Accessed online: 6.28.21.
42. Gender Differences in Time Spent on Parenting and Domestic Responsibilities by High-Achieving Young Physician-Researchers. https://www.ncbi.nlm.nih.gov/pmc/articles/PMC4131769/.
43. Diversity in medicine: Facts and Figures 2019. https://www.aamc.org/data-reports/workforce/report/diversity-medicine-facts-and-figures-2019.
44. These Black women are on the frontlines of the fight against Covid-19. https://www.cnn.com/2021/03/02/us/black-women-covid19-leaders/index.html.
45. Spector ND, Overholser B. COVID-19 and the slide backward for women in academic medicine. JAMA Netw Open. 2020;3(9):–e2021061. https://doi.org/10.1001/jamanetworkopen.2020.21061. Accessed Online: 7.6.2021.
46. COVID-19 Taking a Toll on Med Students, Survey Shows. https://www.medscape.com/viewarticle/939798.
47. AAMC 2020 Physician specialty report https://www.aamc.org/data-reports/workforce/interactive-data/active-physicians-sex-and-specialty-2019, accessed online 8.6.21.
48. Rotbart, H.A., et al. Assessing gender equity in a large academic Department of Pediatrics, Acad Med January 2012. Vol. 87 (1); p 98–104. https://doi.org/10.1097/ACM.0b013e31823be028.
49. Striving for gender equity in academic medicine careers: a call to action. https://pubmed.ncbi.nlm.nih.gov/27332868/. Accessed online: 6.28.21.
50. Assessing gender equity in a large academic department of pediatrics. https://pubmed.ncbi.nlm.nih.gov/22104061/. Accessed online: 6.28.21.
51. Frintner MP, et al. Gender differences in earnings of early- and midcareer Pediatricians. Pediatrics. 2019;144(4)
52. The role of gender and gender equity in The Journal of Pediatrics. https://www.jpeds.com/article/S0022-3476(18)30953-3/abstract. Accessed online: 6.28.21.
53. Gender inequalities on editorial boards of indexed pediatrics journals. https://www.nature.com/articles/s41390-020-01286-5. Accessed online: 6.28.21.
54. Neonatologist salary: factors, equity and gender. https://pubmed.ncbi.nlm.nih.gov/30617285/.
55. Starmer AJ, et al. Gender discrepancies related to Pediatrician work-life balance and household responsibilities. Pediatrics. 2019;144(4):e20182926. https://pediatrics.aappublications.org/content/pediatrics/144/4/e20182926.full.pdf. Accessed online: 6.28.21
56. Spector ND, et al. Women in pediatrics: progress, barriers, and opportunities for equity, diversity, and inclusion. Pediatrics. 2019;144(5):e20192149. https://doi.org/10.1542/peds.2019-2149.
57. Alexander DF, et al. Federation of Pediatric Organizations Task Force on women in Pediatrics: considerations for part-time training and employment for research-intensive fellows and faculty. J Pediatr. 2009;154(1):1–3.
58. Academic Pediatric Association. https://www.academicpeds.org/sig/women-in-medicine/. Accessed online: 9.5.21.
59. https://physiciansfoundation.org/grants/american-academy-of-pediatrics-2/, Accessed Online: 8.6.21.
60. Women In Neonatology. https://services.aap.org/en/community/aap-sections/sonpm/win/about-win/. Accessed online: 9.5.21, Accessed online: 9.5.21.
61. Committee on Pediatric Workforce. https://services.aap.org/en/community/aap-committees/committee-on-pediatric-workforce/. Accessed online: 6.28.21.
62. Women in Pediatric Hospital Medicine. https://www.sohmlibrary.org/women-in-phm.html. Accessed online: 9.5.21.
63. https://www.aps1888.org/diversity-inclusion-codi-committee/; email communication with APS staff, 9/13/21.

64. Advancement, Equity & Leadership for the Women of Pediatric Hospital Medicine. https://www.advancephm.org/. Accessed online 8.6.21.
65. Women in Pediatrics. https://www.womeninpeds.com/about/. Accessed online: 6.28.21.
66. Heisler CA, et al. Has a critical mass of women resulted in gender equity in gynecologic surgery? Am J Obstet Gynecol. 2020;223(5):665–73.
67. Temkin, S. When surgery becomes 'women's work': the devaluationof gynecologic specialties. STAT.. March 12, 2020. https://www.statnews.com/2020/03/12/gynecology-surgical-specialty-devalued-womens-work/ Accessed online 8.6.21.
68. Kowalczyk, L. How a crude photo from a Boston surgeon roiled the medical world. Boston Globe January 11, 2018. https://www.bostonglobe.com/metro/2018/01/11/how-crude-photo-from-boston-surgeon-roiled-medical-world/uPJs9uNW8vauKOvmRZDb2N/story.html. Accessed online: 8.6.21.
69. Baecher-Lind L, et al. A call to action to address gender equity within our specialty: time's up on waiting for change. Obstet Gynecol. 2018;131(6):961–963. 131(6):961–963. https://pubmed.ncbi.nlm.nih.gov/29742671/, Accessed Online:8.6.21.
70. Diversity, Equity & Inclusive Excellence at ACOG. https://www.acog.org/about/diversity-equity-and-inclusive-excellence. Accessed online: 6.28.21.
71. Helitzer DL, et al. Changing the culture of academic medicine: critical mass or critical actors? J Women's Health. 2017:540–8. https://doi.org/10.1089/jwh.2016.6019
72. About the Women's Dermatologic Society (WDS). https://www.womensderm.org/about-wds/history-and-founder.
73. SWIU Value Statement. https://swiu.org/about/past-presidents.aspx.
74. ABOUT AWS. https://www.womensurgeons.org/page/AboutAWS. Accessed online: 6.28.21.
75. American Association for Women in Radiology https://www.aawr.org/ Accessed Online: 9.17.21.
76. Assocation of Women Psychiatrists: History, Mission, Facts. https://associationofwomenpsychiatrists.com/history-mission-facts/. Accessed online: 6.28.21.
77. Ruth Jackson Orthopaedic Society. http://www.rjos.org/index.php/about. Accessed online: 6.28.21.
78. Women in Nephrology https://www.womeninnephrology.org/about/ Accessed Online: 9.17.21.
79. Clem K. A Short History of the American Association of Women Emergency Room Physicians. https://www.acep.org/globalassets/uploads/uploaded-files/acep/membership/sections-of-membership/aawep/briefhistoryofaawep.pdf Accessed Online: 9.17.21.
80. Antonoff MB, et al. Women in thoracic surgery: 30 years of history. Ann Thorac Surg. 2015;101(1):3990409. Jan 1, 2016. https://www.annalsthoracicsurgery.org/article/S0003-4975(15)01863-9/fulltext. Accessed Online: 11.6.21.
81. Women in Neurosurgery. http://www.neurosurgerywins.org/welcome. Accessed Online: 9.17.21.
82. Women in Ophthalmology. https://www.linkedin.com/company/women-in-ophthalmology/about/. Accessed Online: 9–17-21.
83. Korioth T. 10 medical groups form alliance for women's wellness, equity, leadership. AAP News, May 1, 2021. https://www.aappublications.org/news/2021/05/01/fyi-wel050121.
84. AMWA Networking Alliance. https://www.amwa-doc.org/our-work/initiatives/networking-alliance/. Accessed online: 8.6.21.
85. Brodsky L. Sexual Harassment of Physicians: Report 2018. WomenMDResources. June 13,2018. https://www.womenmdresources.com/free-resources/organizations/page/2/. Accessed October 28, 2021
86. Center for women in academic medicine and science. Personal Correspondence, November 2021.

87. Executive Leadership in Academic Medicine® About ELAM. https://drexel.edu/medicine/academics/womens-health-and-leadership/elam/about-elam. Accessed October 28, 2021
88. National Osteopathic Women Physicians Association ByLaws – Midwestern University – Glendale. https://engagemo.atsu.edu/organization/national-osteopathic-women-physicians-organization/documents/view/664200. Accessed October 28, 2021
89. Academy for Women in Academic Emergency Medicine (AWAEM) https://community.saem.org/communities/community-home?CommunityKey=58595efd-f39b-45ac-93b4-398646d11f4f. Accessed October 28, 2021.
90. Advance PHM. Personal Correspondence, November 1, 2021.
91. AAP SOHM PHM. Personal Correspondence, November 6, 2021.
92. Association of Women in Rheumatology LinkedIn. https://www.linkedin.com/company/association-of-women-in-rheumatology/about/. Accessed Online: 9.17.21.
93. FeminEM Personal Correspondence. September 7, 2021.
94. Osborn VW, et al. Society for Women in Radiation Oncology: Residents' perspectives on #MeToo and the founding of SWRO. Applied Radiation Oncology. https://appliedradiation-oncology.com/articles/society-for-women-in-radiation-oncology-residents-perspectives-on-metoo-and-the-founding-of-swro Accessed Online: 9.17.21.
95. WICTA: Women in Cardiothoracic Anesthesia. Newsletter January 2020. https://www.scahq.org/wp-content/uploads/2020/08/wicta-newsletter-JAN2020.pdf. Accessed Online 11.6.21.
96. Women in Anesthesiology. Personal Correspondence, September 7, 2021.
97. Women in Cardiology. Personal Correspondence, October 28, 2021.
98. Women in Emergency Medicine Section of the American Academy of Emergency Medicine. Personal Correspondence, September 17, 2021.
99. Women in Endocrinology. Personal Correspondence, November 3, 2021.
100. Women in Endoscopy. Personal Correspondence, September 2, 2021.
101. American Academy of Otolaryngology-Head and Neck Surgery: Women in Otorhinolaryngology. https://www.entnet.org/get-involved/sections/women-in-otolaryngology. Accessed Online: 9.17.21.
102. Women in Pediatrics. Personal Correspondence, September 17, 2021.
103. Women in Rhinology. Personal Correspondence, October 26, 2021.
104. Women's Neurologists Group (WNG) Personal Correspondence, September 8, 2021.
105. Women in medicine: medical education and networking since 1984. https://womeninmedicine.org. Accessed online October 28, 2021.
106. Eliana Fine, 24: Fighting for Female Physicians. The New York Jewish Week. May 26, 2020. https://jewishweek.timesofisrael.com/eliana-fine. Accessed online October 28, 2021.
107. Collins J. Stronger Together: The Association of Black Women Physicians. Downtown Weekly – The Spirit of Downtown Los Angeles. April 20, 2020. dtla-weekly.com/stronger-together-the-association-of-black-women-physicians. Accessed online October 28, 2021.

Chapter 7
Childbearing, Adoption, Motherhood, and Eldercare by Women in Pediatrics

Laura Chamorro Dauer, Amy Starmer, and Sharon Calaman

Introduction

Women pediatricians assume a wide variety of key roles in their professional and individual lives which evolve significantly through the life course. In this chapter, we will follow a chronologic journey of different life stages: childbearing and adoption to motherhood to eldercare. We will discuss the current state as well as stage-specific barriers and discrepancies which are affecting women in our field at each phase. Ultimately, we will finalize with proposed systemic solutions which we hope to see in the future of pediatrics.

Fertility, Childbearing, and Adoption

> Some argue that women pediatricians work fewer hours per week than male pediatricians and take off months or years for childbearing and caring and therefore do not contribute as much as men. However, it can also be argued that men have more serious illnesses in later

L. C. Dauer
University of Miami Miller School of Medicine, Miami, FL, USA
e-mail: lchamorro@med.miami.edu

A. Starmer
Department of Pediatrics, Boston Children's Hospital, Harvard Medical School, Boston, MA, USA
e-mail: Amy.Starmer@childrens.harvard.edu

S. Calaman (✉)
Department of Pediatrics, Division of Pediatric Critical Care, New York University Grossman School of Medicine, New York, NY, USA
e-mail: Sharon.calaman@NYUlangone.org

N. D. Spector et al. (eds.), *Women in Pediatrics*,
https://doi.org/10.1007/978-3-030-98222-5_7

life and live an average of 2 to 3 years less than women. Therefore, the overall total work hours might not be all that different. In any case, until men can bear children (not likely to happen), this is a moot point. In fact, if women stopped bearing children, there soon would be no need for pediatricians or, in fact, physicians. – Catherine DeAngelis, MD [1].

Fertility

Infertility disproportionately affects women in medicine; this is multifactorial and linked to the nature of our training which is extensive and spans the childbearing years. For women in medicine, the average age of first pregnancy is 30.4 years which is 7.4 years later than the general population. One out of four US women physicians have reported a diagnosis of infertility with an average diagnosis at 33.7 years. Approximately 30% reported diminished ovarian reserve as a cause [2]. Willet et al. examined gender differences among residents' plans to have children during residency and the most influential reasons for these differences. They found that after adjusting for age, institution, postgraduate year, and knowledge of parental leave policies, women were less likely to have children during residency with a threat to career explaining 67% of the gender variance [3]. For various reasons, many women in medicine feel pressure to defer pregnancy during their training, a period which correlates with their peak fertility years. Some of these reasons include stressors intrinsic to training, long hours and night shifts, high to low loan income ratio, and difficulties accessing high-quality childcare. Stentz et al. surveyed 600 women physicians and asked them to reflect on their reproductive and academic decision-making. When asked what they would do differently in retrospect, most respondents (56.8%) would do nothing differently regarding fertility/conception/childbearing, 28.6% would have attempted conception earlier, 17.1% would have gone into a different specialty, and 7.0% would have used cryopreservation to extend fertility [4].

Independent of the cause, it is important to note that infertility is linked to high psychological distress and is also associated with burnout among women in medicine [2]. Fertility coverage has been difficult to obtain with many obstacles in various states except for those few where coverage is legally mandated. Outside of medicine, the culture is changing as private companies such as Starbucks, Bank of America, and Tesla have shifted to include benefit packages which include multiple IVF cycles. However, the healthcare field has been slow to adopt these packages for physicians. As we build toward gender equity, diversity, and inclusion for women in medicine, it is important to bring up the inclusion of comprehensive fertility treatments. Providing comprehensive fertility benefits has been shown to yield improved physical and emotional well-being and job satisfaction, work force recruitment, and employee retention [2]. Comprehensive fertility treatments cultivate a family environment and helps attract and retain talent. These steps pave the way for women in medicine to advance to leadership positions.

The discrepancies and barriers for women in medicine continue from fertility into the childbearing stage. Stentz N et al. examined the level of perceived support for pregnancy at each level of training: before and during medical school, during training, and after training. Physicians who delivered their first child during medical school were significantly less likely to have perceived substantial workplace support than those delivering after completing medical training [4]. It is surprising to see this data as one may suspect residency training to have the lowest level of perceived support given its rigorous nature with long, inflexible work hours. It is important to note this point as we build interventions for women in medicine at each stage. We must take note that structural interventions must start as early as undergraduate medical education.

Childbearing

One thing which strengthens parental support during residency and fellowship training is the delineation of policies by residency programs as suggested by the AAP and ACGME. The pediatric AGCME requirements state that there are circumstances in which residents may be unable to attend work, including parental leave; each program must allow an appropriate length of absence for residents unable to perform their patient care responsibilities and the program must have policies and procedures in place to ensure coverage of patient care; these policies must be implemented without fear of negative consequences for the resident unable to provide clinical work and their fellow residents [5]. The ACGME points are vague and many argue there needs to be specific delineation of guaranteed minimum paid leave that will not require the extension of training [6].

The AAP Parental Leave for Residents and Pediatric Training Programs policy statement requests that pediatric residency programs should have an accessible, written policy for leave to avoid residents having to rely on departmental policies which may not be clear or not relevant for resident training. It delineates that at a minimum parental leave for residents and fellows should conform legally with the Family and Medical Leave Act (FMLA) and respective state laws and meet institutional requirements for ACGME. Regardless of gender, residents who become parents should be guaranteed 6–8 weeks at a minimum of parental leave with pay after the infant's birth. Coparenting, adopting, or fostering of a child should entitle the resident, regardless of gender to the same amount of paid leave as a person who takes maternity/paternity leave. In addition, the American Board of Medical Specialties (ABMS) has established policies requiring its member boards, which include the American Board of Pediatrics, to establish eligibility requirements that allow for at least 6 weeks of parental leave [7].

FMLA requires employers to grant workers up to 12 weeks of annual unpaid leave for the birth or adoption of a child. In order to receive this benefit, an employee must be employed for 12 months which means that residents during their first year of training or first year faculty members would not be eligible for FMLA.

A 2018 JAMA study reviewed childbearing and family leave policies for 15 graduate medical education institutions, and the study found that the average resident duration of childbirth leave was 6.6 weeks [8]. Comparatively, a JAMA 2018 study of academic faculty members at 12 US medical schools found that paid childbearing leave for childbearing mothers was 2 weeks longer with a mean of 8.6 weeks (range of 6–16 weeks) [9]. There is scarce data on average childbirth leave for private pediatricians, but one can infer that given challenges in the private practice world (RVU-based salaries, bonuses, and patient satisfaction score) that private practice pediatricians are not taking the leave they recommend for their patients.

Fertility and Childbearing Next Steps

The AAP has publicly endorsed 12 weeks of paid maternity leave based on the health benefits provided to the child; research in high-income countries show that prolonged parental leave is associated with higher rates of exclusive breastfeeding, on time immunizations, and decreases in neonatal mortality [10–12]. Despite pediatricians being experts in development and understanding the critical parent-child bond in the first 6 months of life, there is a discrepancy between what we recommend to our patients and what we do. However, it is important to highlight that the need for change needs to focus on systemic, institutional change which protect women as early as undergraduate medical education.

Each institution should have written policies with a minimum parental policy which at minimum conform legally with the FMLA state laws. These policies will allow for institutions to be proactive instead of reactive when a pregnancy is announced. Furthermore, written, accessible policies should be widely disseminated by human resource departments to promote early planning which can help reduce anxiety and feelings of guilt by the parent taking leave or any resentment from colleagues for extra work they may need to do in the physician's absence. Most of all given the individual needs of varied pediatric practices (private practice vs academic), it is important for institutional leaders to hold meetings with their faculty to determine the most satisfactory and cost-effective way to provide appropriate coverage during parental leave. This may mean temporary staffing with locum physicians or advanced practice nurses depending on the clinical scenarios. Advance planning may allow for planning to include incentives for physicians who take on additional work during a peer's parental leave. For practices to run smoothly, it is also imperative for the expecting physician to be professional and responsible and notify either the program director or department leadership far in advance when possible, to allow for proper planning. These steps will help cultivate equity in sharing workloads and protect physicians from overly strenuous experiences during their pregnancies which can influence physician wellness and gender equity.

Motherhood

Current State: Challenges and Barriers Faced by Pediatrician Mothers

As pediatrician mothers transition from maternity/family leave and reenter the pediatric workforce, a number of new challenges present themselves. In a recent systematic review of challenges and solutions for physician mothers, Chesak et al. described that these barriers can be organized into individual, organizational/systemic, as well as societal levels [13]. Individually, physician mothers face challenges related to work-life integration, threats to career success, and burnout and mood disorders. Organizational challenges were identified to include a lack of mentorship from and role models who are women to support professional development as well as family leave policies and other policies and/or expectations that affect activities such as breastfeeding, part-time work opportunities, and other expectations surrounding work hours. Finally, on a societal level, factors including gender/sex inequities, maternal discrimination, and challenges related to childcare were noted to reflect society perceptions of physician mothers.

In a related systematic review on the experiences of mothers who are doctors, Hoffman et al. identified three core themes relevant to motherhood and medicine as follows [14]. These themes included the impact of being a doctor on raising children, the impact of being a mother on a medical career, and the strategies and policies that are needed to assist women as they balance motherhood and a medical career.

Regardless of the organizational framework, it is clear that many challenges exist for women pediatricians. In a large cross-sectional nationwide survey of 844 physician mothers, Juengst et al. noted that the most frequently negative experiences when returning to work after family leave as lack of breast pumping facilities (32%), time for breast pumping (48%), difficulty obtaining childcare (35%), and discrimination (18%) [15].

While these national studies have identified important themes relevant to the challenges of motherhood and medicine, the specialty of pediatrics is unique as the majority of early career pediatricians are now women with young children. The American Academy of Pediatrics Pediatrician Life and Career Experience Study (PLACES) is an ongoing longitudinal study monitoring the personal and professional experiences of early and mid-career pediatricians that provides a unique opportunity to examine the perspectives of many pediatrician mothers. While Starmer et al. found that having children was not associated with differences in rates of burnout, work-life balance, or career or life satisfaction, these analyses did not compare these outcomes according to gender [16]. In a companion study, women pediatricians were found to be significantly more likely than male pediatricians to report having primary responsibility for most household responsibilities including routine care of children, cooking, and cleaning. Furthermore, women pediatricians were less satisfied with how responsibilities were shared [17]. PLACES pediatricians participating in the study who have children less than 18 years of age also had a higher odds of always feeling rushed (aOR 2.83, 95% CI 2.05–3.92) [17].

Impact of COVID-19

An important contextual factor that has been shown to increase existing disparities including the challenges faced by pediatrician mothers is the COVID-19 pandemic. A cross-sectional study of 266 physicians in Japan noted that physician mothers demonstrated an increased domestic burden as compared to physician fathers during the pandemic [18]. Specifically, 58% of physician fathers surveyed were from two-income families and had a partner that primarily cared for children, whereas 97% of physician mothers were from two-income families and 95% of the physician mothers reported having to primarily take care of children by themselves. A mixed methods survey of 1806 members of the Physician Moms Group noted that parents with elementary school-aged children frequently raised concerns about homeschooling (44%) and work-life balance (28%), citing qualitative examples of physician mothers who noted, "I'm coming home to a full day of schoolwork after I worked a full day." Additional commentaries and studies noted concern for challenges for women physicians during the pandemic related to decreased academic productivity and compensation, as well as increased mental health and safety concerns such as anxiety and the unknown likelihood of transmission of COVID-19 while breastfeeding [19, 20]. Significant concern has been raised that the family-related care disruptions due to COVID-19 will likely have a profound long-term impact on academic advancement for women working within academic medicine [21].

Solutions and Policies Supporting Pediatrician Mothers

To address and surmount the many challenges and barriers faced by pediatrician mothers both historically and in the context of the COVID-19 pandemic, many strategies and policies have been suggested and trialed to assist women who are working to balance the often-competing demands of a medical career and motherhood. These strategies frequently include mention of the need for policies to expand childcare and breastfeeding facilities. One survey of pediatricians noted that child-friendly workplaces that offered on-site childcare and lactation rooms were considered more likely to be seen as a preferred site for residency training [22]. This notion of having ready access to quality, reliable childcare including off-hours care was identified in multiple additional studies of physician mothers generally as being a key factor to support completion of training as well as career satisfaction [13].

Policies that allow for increased flexibility, such as the inclusion of part-time training options, as well as having increased flexibility in scheduling and call schedules are essential to support pediatrician mothers. In the PLACES study of early and mid-career pediatricians, having advance notification of work schedule was noted to be more likely to be associated with life satisfaction, whereas working in a hectic/chaotic work setting was more likely to be associated with experiencing burnout and lower perceived work-life balance [16].

Mentorship and the support of physician colleagues has also been identified in multiple studies to be a key factor associated with the general well-being and success of pediatrician mothers. Opportunities along these lines include ensuring access to physician mothers as mentors who have demonstrated success at achieving work-life balance as well as implementing facilitated support groups. In a study examining the qualities of ideal mentors, the most common quality was the ability to successfully balance family and full-time practice.

Finally, it is important to note that while policies supporting mentorship, flexibility in work-hours, and access to childcare and breastfeeding support are critical steps toward enhanced support for physician mothers, bias and stigma may still be present that contribute to maternal discrimination [13].

Eldercare

Introduction

An additional challenge for the pediatric workforce is eldercare. By the year 2030, it is projected that 20% of Americans will be 65 or over, exceeding the number of Americans that will be children under 18 [23]. Women pediatricians may be disproportionately affected by this trend. In 2020, the AARP conducted a quantitative study of caregiving. 1392 households were surveyed demonstrating that 16.8% US adults care for someone over 50, up from 14.3% in 2015. Of these caregivers, 61% are women. Women experience caregiving differently as well, increasing the potential demands on them [24]. The 2008 National Study of the Changing Workforce noted that although in their sample men and women were equally likely to have been caregivers, the women provided more regular rather than intermittent care and for more hours per week. Almost half of the women caregivers (46%) were part of the "sandwich generation" caring for children under 18 at home as well [25].

Studies looking at the population at large have demonstrated work impacts for caregivers providing eldercare. The AARP survey in 2020 found that 60% of caregivers were still working and of those 61% experienced some form of a work impact such as going in late or needing to leave early [24]. These types of work impacts have the potential to be even more challenging for physicians as flexibility to adjust one's schedule on short notice is generally lacking with the responsibility to provide clinical coverage and direct patient care. The 2011 National Health and Aging Trends Study found that caregivers providing substantial help, representing 44.1% of caregivers in their sample, were 3x more likely to experience work productivity loss [26].

Current State

Little is published to date about physicians in general as well as pediatricians about the impact of the need to provide eldercare. Much of the literature about women pediatricians focuses on the need to provide childcare and the early career impacts. Templeton, in 2020, surveyed senior women physicians in all disciplines to evaluate their readiness and attitudes toward retirement. Like other data looking at the workforce overall, 20% of the women physicians surveyed were caretakers, with 41% caring for grandchildren, 38% caring for aging parents, and 29% caring for a spouse. Of the group that identified as caretakers, 25% were caring for more than one category [27]. This study suggests that caretaking for women physicians is an issue across the career spectrum, not just for early career practitioners.

Yank et al. conducted a survey of a Physicians Mom's Group on social media, a group with 16,059 members from which there were 5613 responses.16.4% respondents reported additional caregiving responsibilities beyond caring for their children to a friend or family member with a long-term health issue. Of those 48.3% were caring for parents, 16.9% for children or infants, 7.7% for their partners, and 28.6% for other relatives. 16.7% cared for more than one person. Within the 5613 respondents, 989 were pediatricians. Of the 989, 172 (17.3%) had additional caretaking responsibilities, similar to the numbers reported rest of the group. Of note when they compared the group with additional caregiving responsibilities and the group without, while career satisfaction was equivalent, the rates of burnout and mood and anxiety disorders were higher among the women who had additional caregiving responsibilities [28]. Number of hours spent caregiving has been associated with depressive symptoms, with women reporting such symptoms more than men [29]. Wolf reported on data from the 2011 National Health and Aging Trends Study showing that caretakers providing substantial help (44.1% of caretakers in their sample) were at increased risk of emotional difficulty, physical difficulty, and restrictions in participation in valued activities, as well as work productivity loss [26].

In general, combining work and caregiving responsibilities often leads to conflict among the caregivers' work, family, and personal roles [24, 25, 28]. This leaves caregivers at risk for not having adequate energy for any of the roles. For physicians the timing of these demands may come when they are entering mid-late career leading to conflict with leadership positions and continuing on the pathway to promotion. Such demands may result in impediments to women pediatricians being able to take on leadership roles as they may find themselves geographically restricted again as well as needing a more flexible schedule. This may create new barriers for women pediatricians serving in leadership roles even as some of the pipeline issues are addressed.

COVID-19 has exacerbated these time challenges for women. A survey conducted by the National Academies of Sciences, Engineering, and Medicine found women in academic STEMM fields are experiencing increased workload and decreased productivity with the COVID-19 pandemic. The pandemic has exacerbated preexisting gendered division of household labor combined with increased needs for eldercare as well as difficulties with childcare that are disproportionately affecting women. While there have been some institutional accommodations such as extensions on evaluations or grant extensions, these may not be adequate to address the impact on women and may not be exactly what is needed from the institutions at this time to support women, who may need interventions such as a reduced work schedule rather than just extensions. The study calls for further research to prevent STEMM women faculty from falling behind [30].

Solutions

Similar to other challenges around childbearing, workers who are family caregivers in the expressed that what they needed most from the workplace to support them was flexibility in the work schedule – the ability to make schedule changes on short notice, occasional time off during the workday to attend to scheduling needs or appointments, and the ability to either compress one's schedule or work from home. Often, employees expressed that they wished they could access leave time without using vacation first (Table 7.1). One comment that came through in this survey was looking for understanding from management [25]. A commentary highlighted this need for flexibility from a pediatrician viewpoint, noting among the challenges or caring for aging parents being needing to spend time during the workday addressing issues with insurers or financial companies, creating a conflict between the need to make those calls and clinical and scholarly responsibilities [31]. We would anticipate similar themes would emerge from women pediatricians. Eldercare needs to be supported and discussed by leadership to facilitate retention of senior physicians. More study is needed to further explore the impact on women pediatricians.

Table 7.1 Common challenges faced by caregivers and possible solutions

Challenge	Solutions
Need for flexibility to attend appointments, make phone calls during workweek, as well as make schedule changes on short notice	Flexible scheduling such as allowing compression of one's schedule into fewer days or the ability to occasionally work from home
Need for flexibility in vacation time use	Ability to access leave time before vacation days when used for caregiving

Conclusions

Childbearing, motherhood, and eldercare have multiple impacts on women pediatricians that may impact their longitudinal success as well as work-life integration. There are reported impacts on finances. One in five workers providing eldercare report financial hardship [24]. For women pediatricians in general, data from the PLACES study, looking at self-reported earnings from a sample of 1213 early and mid-career pediatricians, demonstrated that women pediatricians were paid less than men. When looking at work-life factors, such as marital status, parental status, choices in work income, or hours for their children, women who had made choices for their children earned significantly less than those who did not, suggesting women are accepting lower salaries for nonmonetary considerations such as flexibility in schedules, fewer hours working, or geographic location [32]. There is impact on the career trajectory for women as well. Carr et al. reported that women faculty with children published less and had less support overall than their male colleagues [33].

Women pediatricians struggle with work-life integration as well. Tawfik looked at work-life integration in physicians and found lower work-life integration in physicians than in the general population, with lower levels in women physicians. Pediatrics was noted to be one of the specialties with the largest gap between men and women [34]. Starmer et al. reported that women pediatricians spend more time on household responsibilities than men [17].

A position paper by the women chairs of AMSPDC identified four areas of focus to improve work-life balance for early career pediatricians as well as to attempt to rectify the balance of women professors in pediatrics. The areas of focus suggested were:

1. The option to work part time – recognizing the need for flexible schedules as the optimal time for childbearing may also be the optimal time for career advancement
2. The need for high-quality childcare availability
3. The integration of flexibility in the physician scientist pathway to allow for "stopping the clock" in the tenure pathways
4. A desire for more women in leadership positions which would link to things like bias training in recruitment and support for formal leadership programs for women [35]

One crucial factor to bear in mind as we look for solutions to address the challenges women pediatricians face as they balance childbearing, motherhood, and eldercare with their career is to avoid solutions that put the burden on the women to fix the issues. McDonald noted the gender bias in literature discussing work-life balance issues, for example, describing how women face "tough choices" in balancing demands of career and family while men were "commendable" when they placed work obligations over home [36]. Often solutions in the literature focus on ways to "educate" women, and encouraging advice like hiring help and prioritizing relationships, without similar recommendations being made for male physicians [36]. Part of moving toward change is challenging these gendered inequities without putting the burden back on women to fix the system, but rather implementing systemic change to allow women the flexibility needed in their schedules as well as the mentorship and leadership opportunities.

References

1. DeAngelis C. Women in pediatrics. JAMA Pediatr. 2015;169(2):106–7.
2. Kaye EC. One in four—the importance of comprehensive fertility benefits for the medical workforce. N Engl J Med. 2020;382(16):1491–3.
3. Willett LL, Wellons MF, Hartig JR, Roenigk L, Panda M, Dearinger AT, Houston TK. Do women residents delay childbearing due to perceived career threats? Acad Med. 2010;85(4):640–6.
4. Stentz NC, Griffith KA, Perkins E, Jones RD, Jagsi R. Fertility and childbearing among American female physicians. J Women's Health. 2016;25(10):1059–65.
5. ACGME Program Requirements for Graduate Medical Education in Pediatrics. Retrieved from https://www.acgme.org/Portals/0/PFAssets/ProgramRequirements/320_Pediatrics_2021v2.pdf?ver=2021-06-24-060023-853.
6. Bressman E. The ACGME Needs to Mandate Parental Leave. 2020. Retrieved from https://blogs.jwatch.org/general-medicine/index.php/2020/01/the-acgme-needs-to-mandate-parental-leave/.
7. American Board of Medical Specialties Policy on Parental, Caregiver and Medical Leave During Training. Retrieved from https://www.abms.org/policies/parental-leave/.
8. Magudia K, Bick A, Cohen J, Ng TS, Weinstein D, Mangurian C, Jagsi R. Childbearing and family leave policies for resident physicians at top training institutions. JAMA. 2018;320(22):2372–4.
9. Riano NS, Linos E, Accurso EC, Sung D, Linos E, Simard JF, Mangurian C. Paid family and childbearing leave policies at top US medical schools. JAMA. 2018;319(6):611–4.
10. Dodson NA, Talib HJ. Paid parental leave for mothers and fathers can improve physician wellness. 2020. Retrieved from https://www.aappublications.org/news/2020/07/01/wellness070120.
11. Heymann J, Sprague AR, Nandi A, Earle A, Batra P, Schickedanz A, Raub A. Paid parental leave and family wellbeing in the sustainable development era. Public Health Rev. 2017;38(1):1–16.
12. Major Pediatric Associations Call for Congressional Action on Paid Leave. 2015. Retrieved from https://www.aap.org/en/news-room/news-releases/aap/2015/familyleaveact/.
13. Chesak SS, Yngve KC, Taylor JM, Voth ER, Bhagra A. Challenges and solutions for physician mothers: a critical review of the literature. Paper presented at the Mayo Clinic Proceedings; 2021.
14. Hoffman R, Mullan J, Nguyen M, Bonney AD. Motherhood and medicine: systematic review of the experiences of mothers who are doctors. Med J Aust. 2020;213(7):329–34.
15. Juengst SB, Royston A, Huang I, Wright B. Family leave and return-to-work experiences of physician mothers. JAMA Netw Open. 2019;2(10):–e1913054.
16. Starmer AJ, Frintner MP, Freed GL. Work–life balance, burnout, and satisfaction of early career pediatricians. Pediatrics. 2016;137(4):1–10.
17. Starmer AJ, Frintner MP, Matos K, Somberg C, Freed G, Byrne BJ. Gender discrepancies related to pediatrician work-life balance and household responsibilities. Pediatrics. 2019;144(4)
18. Nishida S, Nagaishi K, Motoya M, Kumagai A, Terada N, Kasuga A, Miyajima S. Dilemma of physician-mothers faced with an increased home burden and clinical duties in the hospital during the COVID-19 pandemic. PLoS One. 2021;16(6):e0253646.
19. Linos E, Halley MC, Sarkar U, Mangurian C, Sabry H, Olazo K, Linos E. Anxiety levels among physician mothers during the COVID-19 pandemic. Am J Psychiatr. 2021;178(2):203–4.

20. Sarma S, Usmani S. COVID-19 and physician mothers. Acad Med. 2021;96(2):e12–3.
21. Woitowich NC, Jain S, Arora VM, Joffe H. COVID-19 threatens progress toward gender equity within academic medicine. Acad Med. 2021;96(6):813.
22. Berkowitz CD, Frintner MP, Cull WL. Pediatric resident perceptions of family-friendly benefits. Acad Pediatr. 2010;10(5):360–6.
23. Hammer LB, Neal MB. Working sandwiched-generation caregivers: prevalence, characteristics, and outcomes. Psycholog-Manager J. 2008;11(1):93–112. https://doi.org/10.1080/10887150801967324.
24. Caregiving in the US. 2020. Retrieved from https://www.aarp.org/content/dam/aarp/ppi/2020/05/full-report-caregiving-in-the-united-states.doi.10.26419-2Fppi.00103.001.pdf.
25. Aumann K, Galinsky E, Sakai K, Brown M, Bond J. The elder care study: everyday realities and wishes for change. New York: Families and Work Institute; 2010.
26. Wolff JL, Spillman BC, Freedman VA, Kasper JD. A National Profile of family and unpaid caregivers who assist older adults with health care activities. JAMA Intern Med. 2016;176(3):372–9. https://doi.org/10.1001/jamainternmed.2015.7664.
27. Templeton K, Nilsen KM, Walling A. Issues faced by senior women physicians: a National Survey. J Womens Health (Larchmt). 2020;29(7):980–8. https://doi.org/10.1089/jwh.2019.7910.
28. Yank V, Rennels C, Linos E, Choo EK, Jagsi R, Mangurian C. Behavioral health and burnout among physician mothers who care for a person with a serious health problem, long-term illness, or disability. JAMA Intern Med. 2019;179(4):571–4.
29. Cullen JC, Hammer LB, Neal MB, Sinclair RR. Development of a typology of dual-earner couples caring for children and aging parents. J Fam Issues. 2009;30(4):458–83.
30. Dahlberg ML, Higginbotham E. The Impact of COVID-19 on the Careers of Women in Academic Sciences, Engineering, and Medicine. Washington, DC: The National Academies Collection: Reports funded by National Institutes of Health; 2021.
31. Rappaport DI. What caring for my aging parents taught me that medical education did not. JAMA Neurol. 2021;78(1):7–8. https://doi.org/10.1001/jamaneurol.2020.4454.
32. Frintner MP, Sisk B, Byrne BJ, Freed GL, Starmer AJ, Olson LM. Gender differences in earnings of early- and midcareer pediatricians. Pediatrics. 2019;144(4) https://doi.org/10.1542/peds.2018-3955.
33. Carr PL, Ash AS, Friedman RH, Scaramucci A, Barnett RC, Szalacha LE, Moskowitz MA. Relation of family responsibilities and gender to the productivity and career satisfaction of medical faculty. Ann Intern Med. 1998;129(7):532–8.
34. Tawfik DS, Shanafelt TD, Dyrbye LN, Sinsky CA, West CP, Davis AS, Sexton JB. Personal and professional factors associated with work-life integration among US physicians. JAMA Netw Open. 2021;4(5):e2111575. https://doi.org/10.1001/jamanetworkopen.2021.11575.
35. Women Chairs of the Association of Medical School Pediatric Department Chairs. Women in pediatrics: recommendations for the future. Pediatrics. 2007;119(5):1000–5.
36. McDonald J, Chaufan C. Work–life balance in medical practice: the reproduction of patriarchy and the politics of gender. In Underserved and Socially Disadvantaged Groups and Linkages with Health and Health Care Differentials. 2019. p. 205–223.

Part III
Where Do We Go from Here: Achieving Equity and Advancement for Women in the Future

Chapter 8
How Leaders in Pediatrics Can Support Women

Tina L. Cheng and Douglas Carlson

How Leaders Can Support Women

It is well known that women face unique challenges in work, with specific challenges in medicine. As noted in other chapters of this book, women often carry disproportionate home responsibilities, often have lower salaries, and are less represented in promotion and leadership. Sexual harassment unfortunately continues to exist. The disruptions of the COVID-19 pandemic have had a disproportionate effect on women [1]. Recognizing these inequities, there are several ways leaders can act to support the careers of women. We review some of the basics and draw from the sentinel report by the National Academies of Sciences, Engineering, and Medicine on "Sexual Harassment of Women" ([2]) and the article by Narayana et al. [3] focusing on gender equity issues during the pandemic. These recommendations are an excellent framework for institutions and individual leaders.

T. L. Cheng
Department of Pediatrics, University of Cincinnati, Cincinnati Children's Hospital Medical Center, Cincinnati Children's Research Foundation, Cincinnati, OH, USA
e-mail: tina.cheng@cchmc.org

D. Carlson (✉)
Department of Pediatrics, Southern Illinois University School of Medicine, HSHS St. John's Children's Hospital, Springfield, IL, USA
e-mail: dcarlson28@siumed.edu

N. D. Spector et al. (eds.), *Women in Pediatrics*,
https://doi.org/10.1007/978-3-030-98222-5_8

Support for Diversity and Inclusion from Leadership

Clear support from leadership on the importance of diversity, inclusion, and racial and gender equity is essential. The organization's mission, values, and example must recognize that diversity and inclusion enrich our culture, and improve quality of care and quality of ideas. Support and funding need to be aligned with goals of supporting all faculty. This support needs to be explicit. Funding needs to be targeted to increasing diversity and inclusion. Involvement and regular communication with women in medicine groups or women advisory boards should be usual practice to remain abreast of issues and co-create solutions. Ensuring a culture of inclusion involves ensuring a space for women to freely share experiences and support each other and a safe space for disclosing unfair treatment.

Strive for Strong and Diverse Leadership

It is important to publicly state that support of women leaders is among the highest priorities. There is much literature about the dearth of women in leadership and the multiple possible reasons. Diversity and inclusion involve intentional work to overcome implicit biases that exist. This involves inclusion of women in leadership roles and representation on important committees, projects, speaking engagements, and search committees. Open searches for faculty positions should be part of the hiring process to ensure a diversity of candidates. Search committees should undergo implicit bias training and pay attention to the diversity of the candidate pool and finalist lists. Active outreach to candidates is needed to ensure diversity.

Some hiring search committees have ascribed to the Rooney Rule, a 2003 National Football League policy [4] that required teams to interview ethnic minority candidates for head coaching and senior operation jobs. This established an interviewing quota but not a hiring quota. While this is positive to ensure diversity in candidates and finalists, sometimes they are token candidates checking off a box with no chance for the job. This can have the harmful effect of raising expectations and wasting the time of diverse candidates. It can also have the unintended effect of self-doubt among the token candidates who are forever finalists. It is critical that active outreach be combined with sincere consideration for leadership positions.

Create Diverse, Inclusive, and Respectful Environments

Leaders must take purposeful steps to improve cooperation and establish respectful work behavior and healthy inclusive environments. There needs to be an evaluation of all policies and procedures to ensure that opportunities are equal for all and behavioral standards are clear. Changing behaviors is essential. It is more than just saying that gender inequity or harassment is not tolerated. Transparency and accountability on standards of behavior are critical with methods for evaluation and tracking of outcomes. Faculty and staff must be evaluated on professionalism in hiring and promotion. Reporting from individuals cannot be the only method of understanding institutional vulnerabilities. There needs to be routine assessment of culture and climate. There needs to be collaboration among all that oversee faculty and learner work environments.

Ensure Gender Equity in Compensation and Professional Effort

There exists gender inequity in compensation for women in society as a whole, in addition to women in medicine [5, 6]. It is also known that women disproportionally have more uncompensated service-related tasks [7]. Finally, the pandemic may worsen salary disparities because of budgetary tightening and has caused women to leave the workforce [8].

A shortage of women to invite to the table may result in the same women doing a disproportionate amount of committee work resulting in a "minority tax." For instance, women are underrepresented in basic science research. As a result, they often serve on more committees taking them away from their own research. Being a women of color, one of the authors can attest to this double minority tax as she has been on more search committees in her career than most of her peers. While wanting to represent and support the cause, the extra work and opportunity cost are real. It is known that women tend to take on more uncompensated administrative tasks often without leadership titles. Other taxes include handling gender affairs in diversity initiatives, outreach and media to demonstrate diversity, and disproportionate recruitment, retention, and mentoring responsibilities [9]. Acknowledging and "paying" the minority tax should be considered by allowing time for these activities and recognizing their efforts in title and compensation.

Salary reviews for gender equity must be built into institutional systems assessing base salary, call pay, incentive pay, merit pay, and leadership stipends. In addition to equity review when changing an individual salary, periodic comprehensive assessment and correction are critical. Less discussed but also important is standardization and calculation of individual professional effort in areas of clinical care, research, education, and service. This avoids inequity between individuals and raises the visibility and value of important tasks that may need compensated effort in time or salary.

Address the Most Common Form of Sexual Harassment: Gender Harassment

This is harder than it seems. It is much easier to understand and recognize overt sexual coercion and unwanted sexual attention. Verbal and nonverbal behaviors that are subtly insulting, hostile, or degrading are often not easy to spot. There has to be attention to long-standing processes and attitudes to better understand where the problems are and how they can be addressed. Sexual harassment needs to be addressed as a culture and climate issue not just one to meet legal standards (https://www.justice.gov/crt/title-ix). Improving work, education, and training environments needs to be much more than avoidance of legal liability. Institutions can be in compliance with regional, state, and national rules and still be perpetuating unhealthy environments.

There must be support for the reporters of unfair treatment. Reporting issues should always be considered an honorable and courageous action. There should be formal and informal means of recording information about experiences. If reporters are not comfortable filing formal reports, there needs to be a meaningful way to record their experiences informally. Fear of retaliation is a real barrier. Everyone needs to feel comfortable in expressing their concerns.

Strengthen the Pipeline of Women in Science

While there are record numbers of women entering medical school and pediatrics residency, the pipeline of women in science is leaky. Strengthening this pipeline involves ensuring strong supports for women, including strong mentoring teams. Leaders must make sure that junior faculty are connected to committed mentors that address the eight types of or "Cs" of mentors: content mentor, connecting mentor, coaching mentor, cheerleader mentor, critiquing, challenging mentor, career mentor, colleague peer mentor, and clinical mentor [10]. Occasionally, one or two mentors can successfully guide a mentee in all of these "Cs," but often it is a team of mentors. Individuals should reflect on whether their mentoring teams address all of these "Cs." If not, it is critical to actively seek out additional mentorship.

In addition to individualized career development plans and periodic meetings with mentors, leaders should regularly monitor mentoring support and frequency at scheduled evaluations with direct follow-up with identified mentors. Often mentoring relationships are not formalized. In one author's experience, after annual evaluations, she routinely thanks the faculty member's mentors by email for their support. Occasionally, she has heard back from the identified mentor that they did not know they were considered a mentor!

Finally, support and participation in STEM programs for girls early in the pipeline are essential to widen pipeline inflow.

Provide Family Support and Family Friendly Employment Practices and Policies

Leaders in pediatrics should take the lead in ensuring family friendly employment practices and policies. This is critical for the children we serve as well as for our pediatric workforce. These policies should include parental leave for childbirth and adoption that honors time for parents to bond with their new child and also include lactation rooms and schedules that allow breastfeeding time. Available quality childcare including episodic care is a tremendous support for families and increases employee productivity.

Some women may have different trajectories of productivity across their career span with some data showing women having a slower start likely related to child-rearing responsibilities and higher productivity later. Allowing part-time employment often results in high productivity and job satisfaction. Alternate (including remote) and flexible work schedules are important especially in this pandemic time. Promotion policies must allow flexibility for these trajectories and in time clocks at the risk of losing the talent. Additional guidance is available in Chap. 7, "Childbearing, Adoption, Motherhood, and Eldercare by Women in Pediatrics."

Promote Career Development Opportunities

Development and facilitation of women leaders at every level is essential. While women make up nearly half of all US medical students, there are few women in hospital or academic medicine leadership [11]. There needs to be active development of skills in leadership, conflict resolution, mediation, negotiation, and de-escalation and other leadership competencies. Developing a diverse leadership is not passive.

In addition, mentoring, networking, and sponsorship are necessary for academic success. It has been found that the professional networks of women are less extensive compared to male colleagues [12, 13]. A strong mentorship team is critical in academics as described above. Sponsorship and encouraging involvement in national professional organizations are important strategies.

Measure Progress and Conduct Necessary Research

Institutions should work to evaluate and assess efforts to create a more diverse, inclusive, and respectful environment. Formal reports should not be depended upon alone. Data on outcomes in improvements is essential. Information should be shared internally and externally. Not all data will be complimentary to an institution. It is important that everything is shared: improvements, failures, and works in progress.

Research is needed to understand how inequities in opportunities based on gender are perpetuated over time. There should be evaluation of best practices and research on what incentives or deterrents actually help. There needs to be more research about the true levels of sexual misconduct and gender harassment and research to better understand why women are significantly underrepresented in leadership roles in pediatrics and across organized medicine.

Encourage Involvement of Professional Societies and Other Organizations

While most gains will be measured at the level of institutions, it is important that professional societies help accelerate the efforts of members of the organization. Organizations should provide support and guidance for members. National organizations should use their influence to address the issues of gender harassment and gender inequity.

Initiate Legislative Action

Leaders should be concerned beyond their own institutions. Leaders should be advocates for new legislation with the goals of gender equity such as parental leave and protecting all from sexual harassment and other hostile work environments. Related to sexual harassment, it is important to support initiatives such as prohibiting confidentially agreements, banning mandatory arbitration, and making disclosure uniform for all.

Leadership support is essential to achieve gender equity. Continuous improvement involves listening, a culture of inclusion, zero tolerance for gender harassment, equitable policies and procedures, and periodic reassessment.

Personal Stories on the Road to Academic Leadership

Doug Carlson, MD

A few years ago, I received a thank you note from a woman physician that I have deep respect for. In that note, she thanked me for helping sponsor her throughout her career. She wrote the note after attending the Mid-Career Women Faculty Leadership Development Seminar through the Association of American Medical Colleges (AAMC). At the time I was just becoming familiar with the differences between sponsorship and mentorship. I thought, “Why does someone need to thank me for something that is expected of me as a leader?” I reached out to this person to tell her how much I was moved by her thank you note but also to explore my curiosity of the need. Through that point in my career, I believe that I had treated faculty of all genders equally and fairly. In thoughtful retrospect, I am not sure that I had. I cannot think of any specific examples where I have not treated everyone the same, with blindness to gender, but certainly have uncovered implicit biases that I have held through my life and career. I hope that I have removed many of these implicit biases, but it is likely in a few years I will better understand those that still remain today. I have learned that treating everyone the same, giving similar support, or advocating for opportunities is not a passive endeavor. It is something that needs attention in an active, ongoing way.

How does a physician who is a man become recognized as an advocate for women faculty and be referred to as a male ally? I often find it mildly perplexing. I believe it is just treating all faculty the same, but clearly it is more than that. Do I, as a leader, truly treat all faculty the same? Do I give the same opportunities to women and men? Am I more likely to suggest an opportunity for a male colleague than a female colleague with small children? Am I more likely to give a second opportunity than to give someone else a first opportunity? I do believe that while I have always been supportive of women faculty, I may not have been as supportive as possible. I have moved the support of women faculty from something that I believe I did naturally to something that I think about often. While support of women faculty within health care hopefully is coming more naturally, it is clear that we have not yet made all gains needed in support of faculty regardless of gender.

Pediatrics has been a majority women specialty for several decades. Yet we continue to hear that that the issue of gender disparity in leadership positions is one of pipeline. The current state of leadership within pediatrics shows that is more than that. It is not a pipeline issue. At least not the number of women entering the pipeline. When I was a resident in the 1980s, the majority of my colleagues were women. The majority of residents on a national level were women. Yet nearly 40 years later, women are underrepresented in leadership positions in pediatrics. This includes deans, department chairs, and hospital leaders. Why is that? What is underlying, even in pediatrics, which causes disparity in career advancement and salary for the same work?

The causes of disparity of opportunity within pediatrics must be systemic. What are those causes? A couple of years ago I was asked by Judy Schaechter, MD, to be a male colleague on a task force for gender harassment sponsored within the American Association of Medical School Department Pediatric Chairs (AMSPDC). Dr. Schaechter suggested that I read "Consensus Study Report: Sexual Harassment of Women: Climate, Culture and Consequences in Academic Sciences Engineering and Medicine."[2] Even though I am a physician who is a man and is labeled as being an advocate and ally for women physicians, I realized how little I understood. Awareness of the issues based on reading the study and actively trying to get insight has made me more aware of the issues that I had poor understanding of. I thought I understood the issues of sexual harassment. Mostly, I was aware of the potential for issues in regard to the overt types of sexual harassment: unwanted sexual attention or sexual coercion. I rarely saw that, but I also know that it was occurring without me being aware. Without my direct awareness, I felt that I worked in environments that were completely healthy for women. The National Academies of Sciences, Engineering, and Medicine report has made me aware that the overt categories of unwanted sexual attention or sexual coercion are still occurring at a rate far more often than I understood. Most importantly for me was a highlighting of the concept of gender harassment. Gender harassment is the most common type of sexual harassment. As defined by Fitzgerald, Gelfand, and Drasgow, gender harassment is a "broad range of verbal and nonverbal behaviors not aimed at sexual coercion but that convey insulting hostile and degrading attitudes about members of one gender" [14]. I did not fully understand the impact of this type of sexual harassment. Implicit gender harassment by institutions and individuals likely has a large role in the underrepresentation of women in leadership positions within pediatrics and medicine broadly.

As I look at my career, there are some facts that I find distressing. Not in things that I overtly did or inadvertently did not do but in review of the history of institutions that I have deep gratitude and respect for. I have never had a woman boss. I certainly have worked with women in more senior leadership roles than mine – hospital president and chief clinical officer – but never someone that I directly reported to. I did not seek that out as opportunities arose but the fact that I have never had a woman direct supervisor in a 35-year career in pediatrics is telling. When I started as the Chair of my current department, there had been one woman full professor in the history of the department. I am working to correct that, but still women are significantly underrepresented at the professor level. There have been five chairs in the 50-year history of my current department, all white men. At my previous medical school, there have only been white male Chairs of the Department of Pediatrics in over 100 years. Does this make my Department of Pediatrics guilty of not supporting women faculty as well as we should have? I think it does. The issue is hard to trace back to individuals. I believe it is the little decisions that were made in hiring, support, sponsorship, mentorship, and promotion that have all added up to get us where we are. We need to do better at all levels: support of individuals, changing local institutions, and changing national attitudes. There is no one-step solution. Solutions are complex and need to come from all of us.

It is important for leaders to support all that report to them in their career development. It is important to develop a welcoming environment where all can thrive. It is important for leaders to understand the institutional biases that may disproportionately affect diverse groups of developing leaders. Setting the proper environment that leads to equitable opportunities is not passive. It is an active pursuit that needs to be reviewed often. I am honored whenever anyone refers to me as a leader that understands the issues of my women co-workers, a leader that provides support for all. I am not sure that I deserve this recognition, but I am on a journey to appreciate, advocate, and elevate women to the best of my ability.

Tina Cheng, MD, MPH

I owe a debt of gratitude to all the women before me who have paved the way. The first was my mother, a Chinese immigrant who faced many obstacles but had a long career as a kindergarten teacher. My father was a biochemistry researcher. It was no wonder then that their daughter became an academic pediatrician merging both of their occupations. As the middle of three sisters, my parents instilled in us that we could achieve anything that we set our minds to, regardless of gender. Though it was thought to be "unlucky" to have three daughters, my parents valued education and set high expectations for us to excel in our chosen fields and do good.

Born in Toledo, Ohio, I grew up in Coralville, Iowa, where I wanted to become a doctor starting in grade school. My parents kept a School Days book that documented each year of my primary schooling (Fig. 8.1). It is notable that my School Days book had a section on "when I grow up, I want to be…." The choices were divided by gender. Boys could choose from fireman, policeman, cowboy, astronaut,

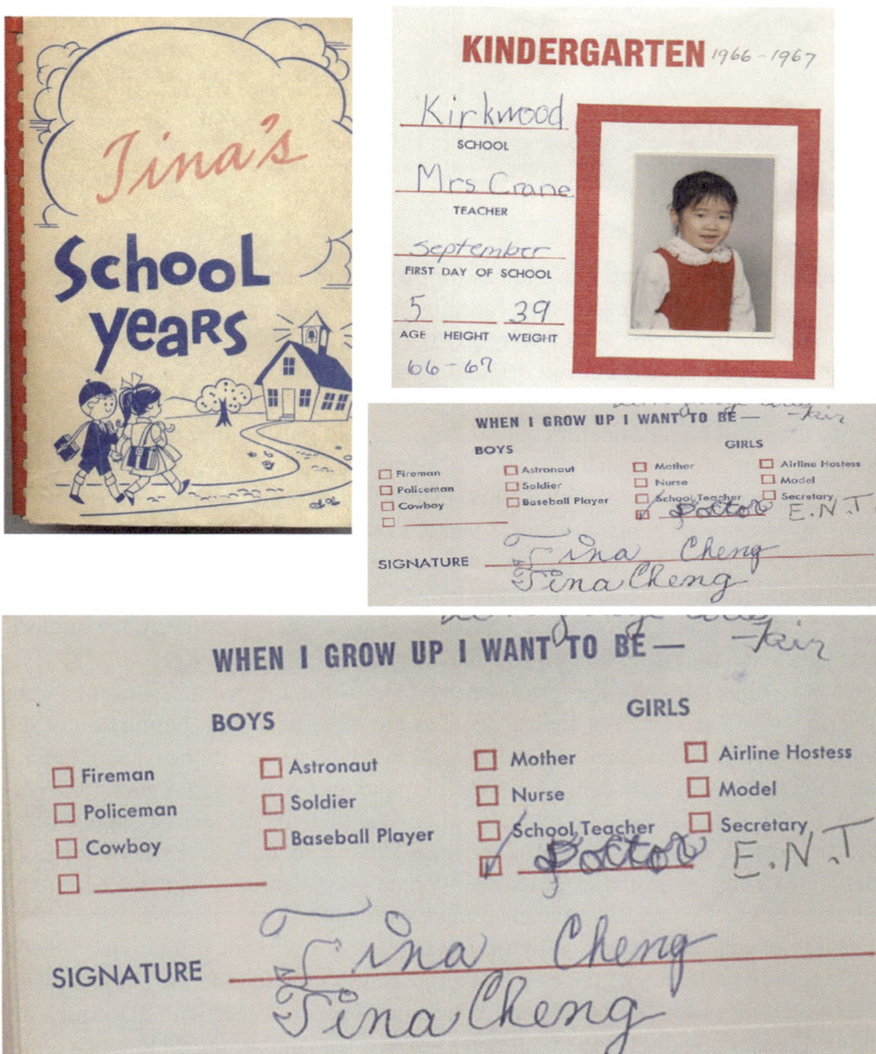

Fig. 8.1 Photo of Tina Cheng's childhood "School Years" book, 1966–1967

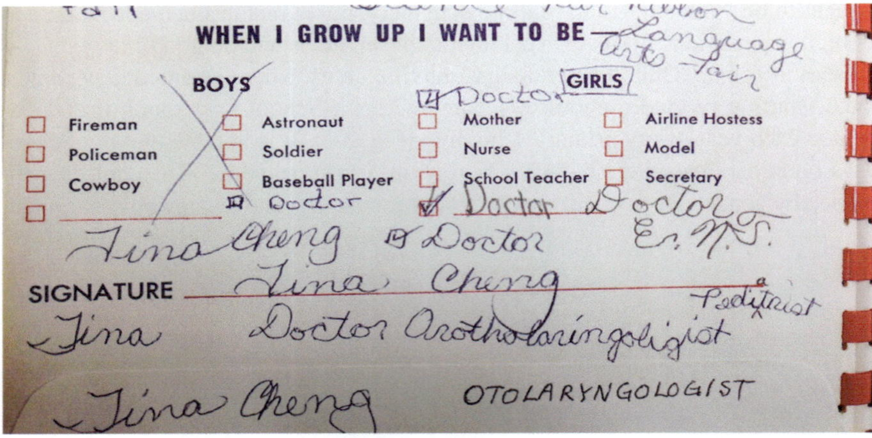

Fig. 8.1 (continued)

soldier, or baseball player. The choices for girls were mother, nurse, schoolteacher, airline hostess, model, or secretary. Starting in kindergarten, I filled out the "other" box and wrote in "doctor, ENT." Why an ENT? I had frequent nosebleeds as a child. I went to several physicians and decided I wanted to help other children by being a doctor.

My dream of being a doctor continued throughout my childhood. Unfortunately, there are too many children today, and too many women, who aren't taught to dream or do not have circumstances that allow them to reach their dreams. When I would share my dreams of being a doctor, I was told, "Hmmm, well pediatrics is a good field for a woman." This increased my desire to succeed. Unfortunately, it also made me discount going into pediatrics early on.

While my medical school class was over a third women, there were few minorities. Our anatomy professor showed Playboy centerfolds during class. While this itself was objectionable, the reactions by others that the women students were "oversensitive" and "what's the big deal?" were more upsetting. Discussion of the impact of social determinants of health and health disparities by race and ethnicity was rare. There was little diversity in teaching pictures with the exception of depictions of all dark-skinned individuals when learning about sexually transmitted infections. My medical school experience led me to co-found the Women In Medicine Group and American Medical Women's Association Chapter. It also reaffirmed my career commitment to ensuring health equity.

While pediatrics was not really on my list going into clinical rotations, I loved working with children and realized that children were the foundation of health with great potential to for lasting impact. While I enjoyed working with adult patients and had great empathy for their challenges, I saw real opportunities to make a difference working earlier in the life course.

As a woman physician in my residency and throughout my career, I was often mistaken for a nurse. As one of two Asian women in my residency class, we were often thought to be the same person. The number of times I was called her name, and vice versa, was too numerous to count.

Because of my interest in individual and population health, following chief residency, I pursued a Master's in Public Health Degree at UC, Berkeley, and a Preventive Medicine Residency. I then moved to the east coast for a fellowship in Academic Pediatrics focused on research followed by my first academic job at Children's National Medical Center. My first child was born during fellowship and at the time I was unsure how academics and research would meld with family life. I soon learned that research was a creative outlet, provided autonomy to focus on my scholarship and family, and offered an important path to improve child health practice and policy. I was able to attend many of my children's events because of the autonomy provided by academic time. Writing grants and manuscripts occurred around my family's schedule. I always had reading available while waiting for soccer practice completion. A natural early bird, work was often completed prior to my family's wakening.

Today, I show trainees my publication trajectory over time demonstrating slight downturns after the births of my two children but with acceleration in time. I was fortunate to have healthy children, the salary of a physician, and supports including a husband with a more flexible schedule, and a long-term wonderful babysitter.

Early in my career, I was offered leadership opportunities, and I almost always said yes. It started when I was asked to be nominated as the Accreditation Council on Graduate Medical Education Pediatrics Residency Review Committee Resident Representative. I was fortunate to be selected and had the opportunity to meet luminaries in pediatrics. It was a lot of work between my every third night call schedule but well worth it. Through that experience, doors opened. I co-founded the American Academy of Pediatrics (AAP) Resident Section and served as the resident representative on several AAP committees. Often the youngest and among a minority of women, I learned from so many leaders in pediatrics, realized the power of these professional organizations in shaping practice and policy, and slowly found my voice. Mentorship was a critical factor in my development and I was, and continue to have, wonderful, mostly mentors who are men at each stage of my career, many who have remained lifetime mentors.

Seven years into my position at the Children's National Medical Center, I was promoted to Associate Professor and was called to look at a Division Director job at Johns Hopkins University. I was unsure if it was the right time to become a Division Director and my mentor told me that "looking can be dangerous." Nonetheless, I entered the danger and ended up moving to Johns Hopkins University as the Division Director of General Pediatrics and Adolescent Medicine. My daughter was 8 years old at the time and I told her this new job would involve being the boss of more people. When I asked her, "Do you think I could do this?" she didn't skip a beat and responded, "I can teach you!"

Amid the academic environment at Hopkins, my career flourished, and more opportunities came for leadership at Johns Hopkins and in professional organizations. In the history of Johns Hopkins University School of Medicine, I became only the 138th woman professor in 2008. I have asked what the number is for men and have been told it is not counted. I went on to become the Chair of Pediatrics and Pediatrician-In-Chief in 2016, only one of two women and one of three persons of color (one African American, two Asians) among the 21 clinical Department Chairs at Johns Hopkins University. I went on to become Chair of Pediatrics, Chief Medical Officer, and Director of the Cincinnati Children's Research Foundation to focus on children. While there are more women in pediatrics, there continue to be unique issues for women in academia including a dearth of women leaders. While there has been progress since the time Playboy pin-ups were tolerated in medical education, there is still much work to do.

My clinical, educational, and research career has focused on health equity and how we can stimulate young people who may not have the same opportunities as I did, to dream big and to have the possibility to achieve their dreams. It has taken a pandemic and a video of a murder to raise the country's consciousness about the urgent need for equity and social justice. I believe diversity and inclusion enriches all of us and improves our missions in clinical care, education, and research. We need to lead the way for the next generation.

References

1. Jagsi R, Fuentes-Afflick E, Higginbotham E. Promoting equity for women in medicine: seizing a disruptive opportunity. NEJM. 2021;384(24):2265–7.
2. National Academies of Sciences, Engineering and Medicine. Sexual harassment of women: climate, culture, and consequences in Academic Sciences, engineering, and medicine. Washington, DC: The National Academies Press; 2018. https://doi.org/10.17226/24994
3. Narayana S, Roy B, Merriam S, et al. Minding the gap: organizational strategies to promote gender equity in academic medicine during the COVID-19 pandemic. J Gen Intern Med. 2020;35(12):3681–4.
4. Collins BW. Tackling unconscious bias in hiring practices: the plight of the Rooney rule. N Y Univ Law Rev. 2007;82(3):870–912. ISSN 0028-7881
5. Dander VM, Lautenberger DM. Exploring faculty salary equity at U.S. medical schools by gender and race/ethnicity. Washington, DC: AAMC; 2021.
6. Spector ND, Asante PA, Marcelin JR, Poorman JA, Larson AR, Salles A, Oxentenko AS, Silver JK. Women in pediatrics: progress, barriers, and opportunities for equity, diversity, and inclusion. Pediatrics. 2019;144(5):e20192149.
7. Babcock L, Recalde MP, Verterlund L. Why women volunteer for tasks that don't lead to promotions. Harvard Business Review. Published July 16, 2018. https://hbr.org/2018/07/why-women-volunteer-for-tasks-that-dont-lead-to-promotions. Accessed October 5, 2021.
8. National Academies of Sciences, Engineering and Medicine. The impact of COVID-19 on the careers of women in Academic Sciences, engineering and medicine. Washington, DC: The National Academies Press; 2021. https://doi.org/10.17226/26061
9. Williamson T, Goodwin CR, Ubel PA. Minority tax reform: avoiding overtaxing minorities when we need them most. New Engl J Med. 2021;384(20):1877–9. https://www.justice.gov/crt/title-ix. Accessed October 11, 2021.
10. Cheng TL, Hackworth JM. The "C's" of mentoring: using adult learning theory and the right mentors to position early-career investigators for success. J Pediatr. 2021;20:S0022-3476(21)00261-4.

11. Mangurian C, Linos E, Sarkar U, Rodriguez C, Jagsi R. What's holding women in medicine back from leadership? Harvard Business Review. Published June 19, 2018, rev Nov 7, 2018. Available at: https://hbr.org/2018/06/whats-holding-women-in-medicine-back-from-leadership#:~:text=What's%20Holding%20Women%20Back,promoted%20because%20of%20their%20gender. Accessed October 5, 2021.
12. Hitchcock M, Bland CJ, Hekelman FP, Blumenthal MG. Professional networks: the influence of colleagues on the academic success of faculty. Acad Med. 1995;70(12):1108–16.
13. Uzzi B. Men and women need different kinds of networks to succeed. Harvard Business Review. Published Feb 25, 2019. Available at: https://hbr.org/2019/02/research-men-and-women-need-different-kinds-of-networks-to-succeed. Accessed October 5, 2021.
14. Fitzgerald LF, Gelfand MJ, Drasgow F. Measuring sexual harassment: theoretical and psychometric advances. Basic Appl Soc Psychol. 1995;17(4):425–45. https://doi.org/10.1207/s15324834basp1704_2.

Chapter 9
A Step-Wise Approach to Equity: Implementing Effective Policies and Programs in Pediatrics

Erin E. Shaughnessy and Vineeta Mittal

Disparities for women in pediatrics have existed for decades [1–8]. The term "equal opportunity" has been used to describe ongoing commitment to equal treatment by organizations despite the inequity in pay, promotion, leadership, and rank that women in medicine have encountered for years. Recent publications highlight inequity in every aspect of medical careers for women [1–10].

In pediatrics, women comprise 72.3% of residents, 63.3% of practicing physicians, and 57.4% of academicians, yet women comprise of only 16.8% of deans and 18% of medical school department chairs and 26.2% of pediatric chairs [8–11]. Despite an increase in percentage of women as professors to 25%, the number of women as deans has remained steady since 2016 [10–12]. One would assume that pediatrics with its high proportion of women in the workforce would lead the way with higher number of executive and senior leaders compared to other medical and surgical fields. But women of all backgrounds and specialty types experience similar disparities in the workplace and in achieving executive leadership roles that involve handling and controlling resources [1]. Women in pediatrics face similar challenges related to work-life integration, workplace culture, climate, disparity in compensation, rank, promotions, harassment, microaggression, and implicit biases [1]. Challenges of intersectionality, that is, multiple underrepresented identities including gender, race, sexual orientation, ability, age, or socioeconomic status, further complicate the advancement of underrepresented women [1, 13]. These disparities are being acknowledged and called out by a few national pediatric organizations.

E. E. Shaughnessy (✉)
Department of Pediatrics, University of Alabama at Birmingham, Birmingham, AL, USA
e-mail: eshaughnessy@uabmc.edu

V. Mittal
Department of Pediatrics, UTSW Medical Center & Children's Health, Dallas, TX, USA
e-mail: Vineeta.Mittal@utsouthwestern.edu

N. D. Spector et al. (eds.), *Women in Pediatrics*,
https://doi.org/10.1007/978-3-030-98222-5_9

In 2018, the Women's Wellness through Equity and Leadership (WEL) project, led by the American Academy of Pediatrics (AAP) and in collaboration with the American Academy of Family Physicians (AAFP), American College of Obstetricians and Gynecologists (ACOG), American College of Physicians (ACP), American Hospital Association (AHA), and American Psychiatric Association (APA), brought together a diverse group of women physicians to empower them to build cross-specialty relationships critical to address the myriad of issues facing physicians in the evolving US healthcare system [14]. The project identified many of the current challenges that women face and explored strategies for advancing women in medicine [14]. In 2019, Spector et al. [2] identified that fair treatment of women in pediatrics will require commitment from four key gatekeepers groups: academic medical centers, hospitals, healthcare organizations, and practices, medical societies, journals, and funding agencies. They further described a six-step equity, diversity, and inclusion cycle through a scientific and data-driven approach that would pave the path forward for women in medicine (Fig. 9.1) [2].

The current culture of inequity, gender bias, and discrimination for women in medicine is pervasive. Such a pervasive culture leads to burnout for women and favors men over women. It promotes inequity in pay, promotion, and leadership. A drastic change is needed. But where will the change come from and how will the change be implemented and measured? Literature shows that women physicians achieve better patient outcomes; a diverse workforce has also been shown to achieve better healthcare outcomes and reduce disparities in care [15, 16]. Whether change is top-down, bottom-up, or mandated through national organizations, it will require thoughtful and strategic implementation.

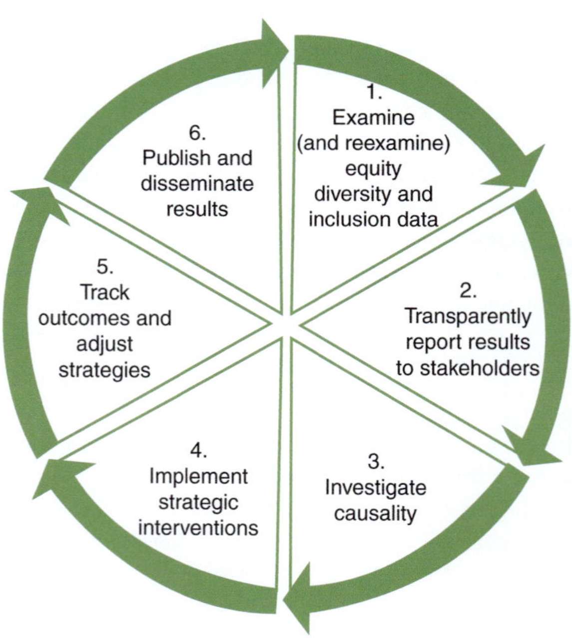

Fig. 9.1 The equity, diversity, and inclusion cycle: a strategic approach to accountable documentation and the resolution of gender (and other) disparities in medicine [1]

This chapter aims to identify the key steps that organizations must take to implement, measure, and manage change related to global issues faced by women in pediatrics, and to successfully advance, promote, recruit, and retain women in pediatrics. We adapted the time-tested change management framework by John Kotter [1] and Nancy Spector et al.'s equity, diversity, and inclusion cycle [2] to create this stepwise approach.

Box: Stepwise Approach to Drive Equity in the Pediatric Workplace

Step 1: Acknowledge the problem and commit to change
Step 2: Create a powerful coalition
Step 3: Create and communicate a vision for change
Step 4: Develop strategic plan using improvement science and empower others to act
Step 5. Develop quick wins and build on change
Step 6. Ensure sustainability and institutionalize change

A Stepwise Approach to Drive Equity in Pediatric Workplace

Step 1: Acknowledge the Problem and Commit to Change

Implementing change in any organization first requires acknowledging the problem and committing to change. Leaders of institutions can recognize pressing problems as opportunities and start by transparently acknowledging the current organizational problem(s) and commit to change. Sharing the most recent organizational data elements (such as in Table 9.1) in open forums and committing to change is the first step in engaging faculty.

Table 9.1 Initial overview of organizational culture: metrics by gender and URiM[a] status

Proposed metrics, reported as overall numbers and proportion by gender and URiM status
Proportion of faculty
Proportion by academic rank
Average time to promotion in years
Total compensation (by year of experience vs benchmark)
Percentage of leadership positions occupied by women and URiM
Total compensation among leaders
Organizational awards (nominations, awards)
Grand rounds invitations
Representation in committees

[a] URiM: underrepresented in medicine

Step 2: Create a Powerful Coalition

Form a multidisciplinary and equitable coalition of leaders within the institution who can persuade others to implement policies and procedures for change. Organizations can do so by establishing an "Office of Equity" or an equity taskforce for change management. Such a powerful coalition should represent a broad group of faculty that are diverse in age, gender, race and ethnicity, rank, and power structure. Such a coalition can be charged to review literature and internal data and develop a vision and strategic plan.

Step 3: Create and Communicate a Vision for Change

The third step is to create a vision and a strategic plan to initiate change. It is crucial that organizations review gender- and URiM-specific internal data and develop a clear vision for change including a strategic plan for stepwise approach to change. Examining (and re-examining) gender and URiM data can help identify early wins (e.g., equity in pay/promotion/committees). Once the vision is established, then it should be shared broadly in a transparent manner.

Step 4: Develop Strategic Plan Using Improvement Science and Empower Others to Act

While the first step is acknowledging the problem and committing to change, equally important are identifying key strategic initiatives required for change. Internal data can identify and drive these initiatives (Table 9.1). Once the priorities are identified, writing and communicating SMART aims, which are specific, measurable, attainable, realistic, and time-bound [17], is important. These goals clearly define a population (i.e., pediatric practice), a metric, and a timeline, and are ambitious enough to be worthy of effort but also clearly achievable. As each strategic priority is identified, organizations will benefit from writing SMART aims and developing key driver diagrams to identify drivers and interventions required for change. Sharing the strategic plan, with clear metrics and timeline for achievement, will ensure accountability and demonstrate commitment.

For example, a global aim may be to achieve equity in academic promotion for women and men. To work toward this vision, a SMART aim might be to "increase the percentage of women promoted to professor within 8 years of associate professor rank by 20% within 3 years." Writing a data-driven SMART aim requires some investigation into the current state of the problem at the organization to target the issue and identify an achievable, but worthy, goal.

Once goals are defined, the next step is to generate a hypothesis as to key drivers [19]. What do organizational leaders believe are the factors which most influence the issue? Key drivers are important because they inform the HOW of change. They define the organization's theory of successful change. How might an organization refine what may be a long list of potential drivers? Published literature, local data, stakeholder opinions, and knowledge of an organization's climate and culture (including appetite for change) can drive these. For example, the key driver diagram for improving timely academic promotion for women in pediatrics may have many potential key drivers as per Fig. 9.2: clear, objective promotion criteria, equitable process for inviting speakers to institutional conferences, implementation of mentorship programs, term limits for key committee positions, and changes in process for institutional grant review scoring rubric to emphasize science rather than investigator background.

How will the leaders of this work know where to focus? Review of internal quantitative data (such as internal grant awards to women vs men, time to promotion, mentorship and sponsorship opportunities, leadership opportunities, and involvement in committees) may be helpful. Qualitative data from faculty interviews, surveys, or focus groups may elucidate what faculty perceive as the biggest barrier. An example of survey data in helping focus an intervention is displayed in Fig. 9.3. The figure shows a possible Pareto diagram generated by a survey of women faculty who are 5 or more years into assistant professor rank, with the diagram showing the frequency of response to "select what you perceive to be the most significant barrier to promotion to associate professor." Pareto diagrams are powerful because the Pareto principle holds that 20% of the causes are typically responsible for 80% of the effect. Therefore, targeting the 20% of causes (drivers) will help drive the largest change [18].

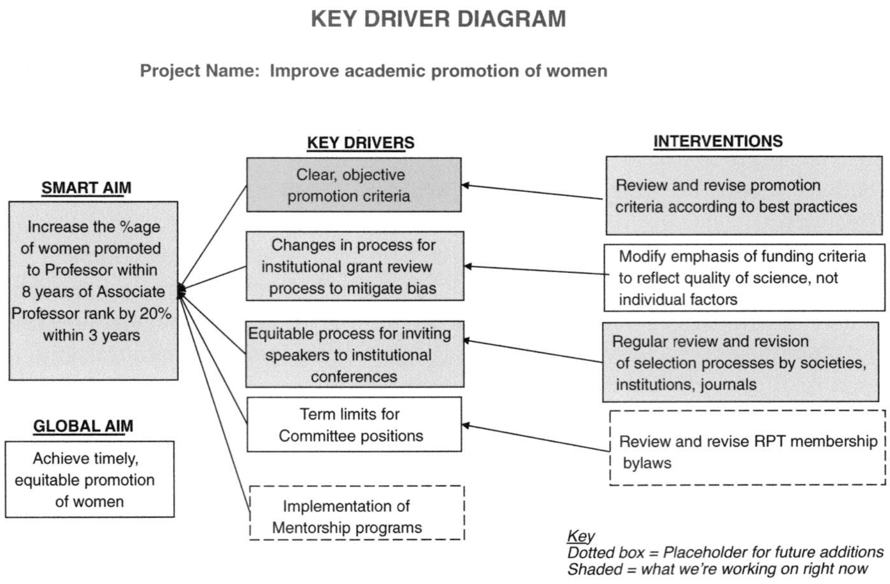

Fig. 9.2 Key driver diagram for an initiative to improve the timely and equitable promotion of women

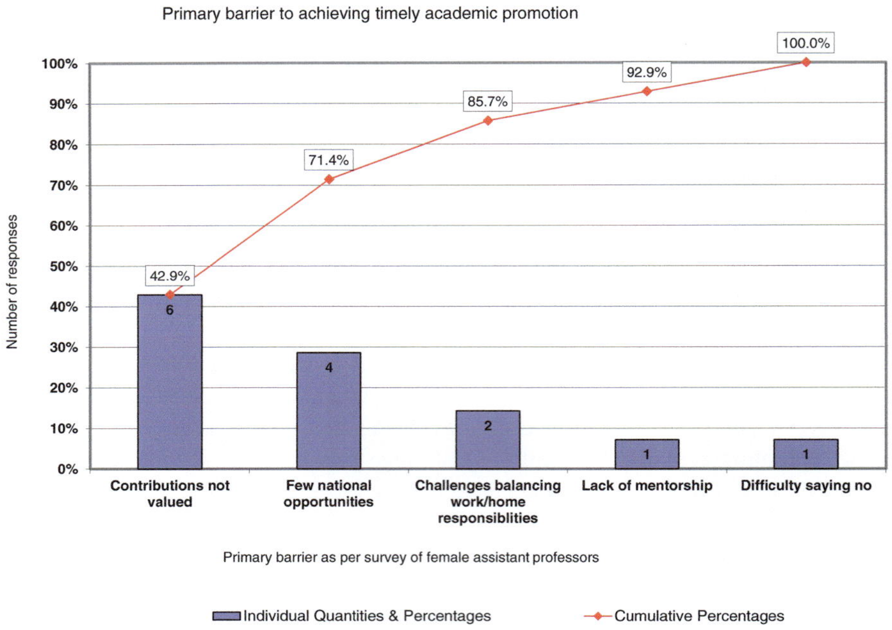

Fig. 9.3 Pareto diagram of responses to a survey of female assistant professors regarding the primary barrier to achieving timely academic promotion

What other data might be useful? Perhaps the decision-makers on nominating faculty for promotion (division directors, department chairs) and those reviewing packets (i.e., promotions committees) could be asked to provide feedback on why faculty were not deemed "ready." This source of data may illuminate different key drivers (Fig. 9.4).

Once key drivers are chosen, the next step is to brainstorm interventions involving a larger group that includes both men and women in pediatrics. Potential interventions should be tested on a small scale and data collected on feasibility, effectiveness, and any untoward effect (i.e., balancing measure). Interventions promising on a small scale can then be scaled up and spread to increase impact.

An example potential intervention to impact timely academic promotion might be the introduction of career development committees for faculty at regular intervals in a promotion cycle. Instead of mandating career development committees as policy, a small group of faculty could be chosen as a pilot group, and the logistics of selecting, scheduling, and running a career development committee could be worked out on a small scale, with data collected on usefulness/value. Data from the pilot group could then be used to "scale up" the availability of career development committees in a way that maximizes efficacy.

It bears noting that having faculty engagement in the early intervention planning will not only help improve the intervention but will also help with buy-in and acceptability to a larger number of faculty.

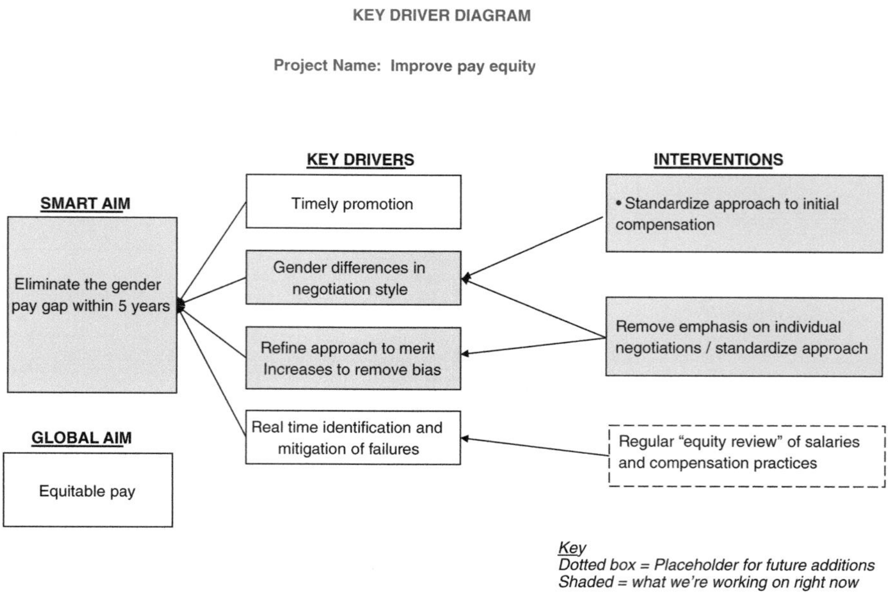

Fig. 9.4 Key driver diagram for an initiative to achieve equitable pay

To help jump-start an organization's approach to this important quality improvement, we provide three additional common disparities with suggested aims, key drivers, and potential interventions.

1. Improve pay equity. One key driver is gender-driven differences in negotiation styles. Women have been socialized to be less assertive than men when asking for compensation, and are in a double bind in that they are also perceived to be more aggressive when asking for resources, while men are perceived as more confident and competent in asking for the same [20]. How can organizations help women avoid this trap? A simple answer is to move away from individual negotiations and toward a more standard approach, especially for entry-level positions where standardization is more possible. Another potential intervention may be performing regular equity reviews, whereby the compensation for faculty in similar roles and rank is reviewed and adjustments are made to achieve equity (Fig. 9.4).
2. Improve representation of women in senior leadership roles. One key driver that may be common to many organizations is the tendency to ask women to serve on committees and in roles that do not control resources rather than those that do allocate resources. We label this tension "service vs power." A common example is women serving in educational roles and social or wellness committees (service roles), rather than chairing finance or compensation committees (power roles) (Fig. 9.5).
3. Improve inclusive, supportive environment. This key driver diagram illustrates that organizations can harness tools used for other key mission-driven efforts,

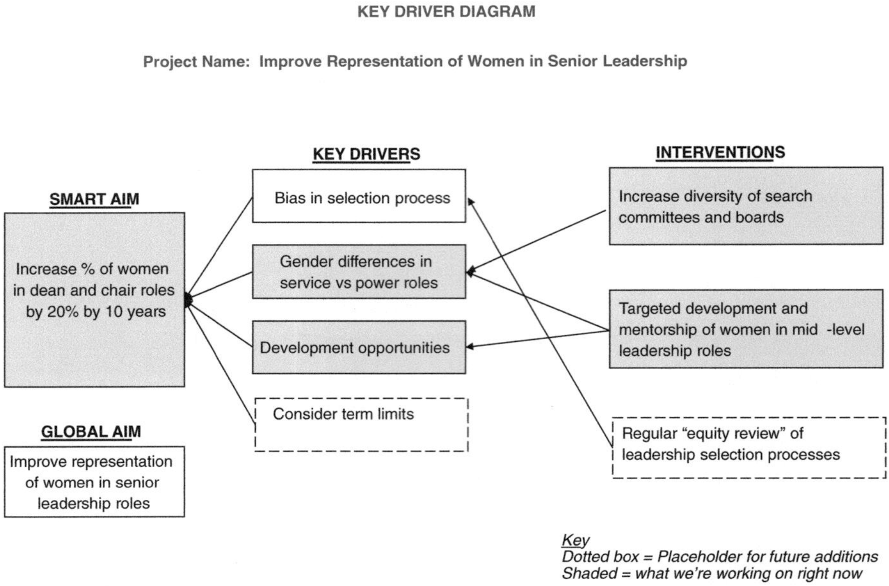

Fig. 9.5 Key driver diagram for an initiative to improve representation of women in senior leadership roles

such as improving patient safety, to inform work to improve an inclusive, nonhierarchical culture. For example, many children's hospitals administer a safety culture survey every 1–2 years to assess progress in safety culture. This instrument measures attitudes and behaviors that are also foundational to inclusion and thus can be used to inform diversity, equity, and inclusion efforts as well (Fig. 9.6).

Step 5: Develop Quick Wins and Build on Change

It is important to celebrate small wins and build momentum for change. Announcing a diverse taskforce or sharing data with proposed outcomes measures can be an example of developing quick wins. Sharing such early wins with all stakeholders including frontline physicians can further help build on the change by improving buy-in, building trust and accountability. To maintain trust, continuing to share progress and timeline is equally important.

Effective communication and transparency around reporting data for equity efforts is important for several reasons. Reporting data via published dashboards or other easily accessible and visible routes communicates the organization's commitment to equity, promotes an accountable and equitable culture, and keeps all levels of the organization informed of progress and challenges. It moves equity from a bullet point in the mission statement into a visible effort toward meaningful change.

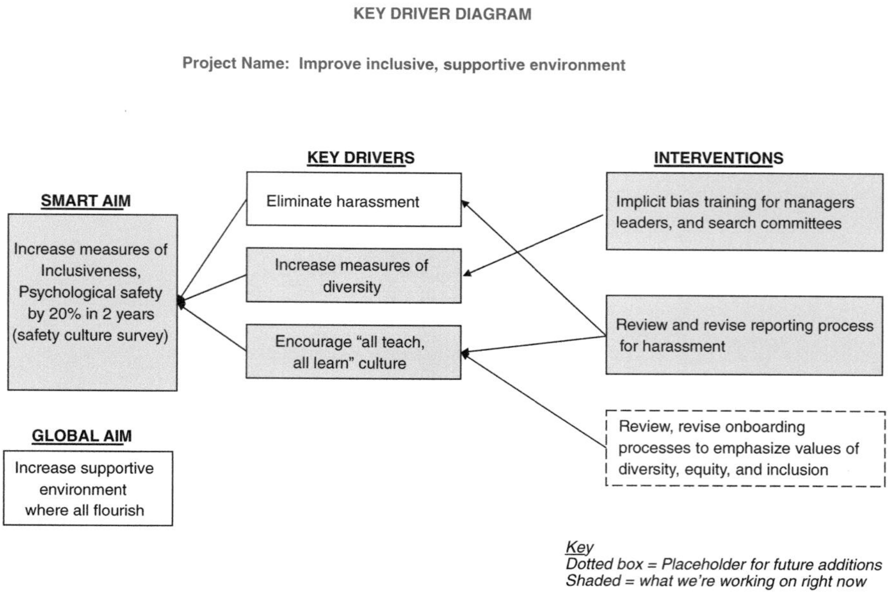

Fig. 9.6 Key driver diagram for a project to achieve an inclusive environment

Step 6: Ensure Sustainability and Institutionalize Change

A challenge that is common to all quality improvement work is sustaining progress once a project moves from an active improvement phase to one of sustaining success. Once attention moves to another initiative, it can be easy for progress to backslide. One way to guard against this tendency is to maintain key indicator measures on a dashboard. With data reported on a regular basis, leaders can see if previous gains are faltering. After making significant progress toward pay equity, one institution (University of Alabama at Birmingham Department of Pediatrics) has implemented an annual "compensation equity review" process to guard against pay inequity for women and underrepresented groups. Mitigating emerging disparities on an annual basis can thus prevent large inequities from recurring.

Identify Policies and Programs for Achieving Gender Equity Milestones

While we provided key driver diagrams for key initiatives, organizations must review current policies and procedures and revise old policies or develop new policies. Some of the policies and programs that are crucial for equity include those in Table 9.2. Such policies should be reviewed on a regular agreed upon interval, be revised regularly, and be available to all faculty.

Table 9.2 Suggested areas for policies/procedures with sample resources

Programs that support progress for women in pediatrics	WEL initiative (https://drexel.edu/medicine/academics/womens-health-and-leadership/elam/blog/womens-wellness-through-equity-and-leadership-project/) ADVANCE PHM (www.advancephm.org/) FeminEM (feminem.org/) ELAM (https://drexel.edu/medicine/academics/womens-health-and-leadership/elam/)
Policy to handle harassment or discrimination complaints	Title IX office at your institution
Promotion criteria that value DEI work	Revised promotion criteria at Harvard Medical School (https://fa.hms.harvard.edu/promotion-profile-library)
Academic journal policies	*Journal of Hospital Medicine* https://www.journalofhospitalmedicine.com/jhospmed/article/227669/hospital-medicine/promoting-gender-equity-journal-hospital-medicine
Progressive FMLA policies	Business Insider's best parental leave policies https://www.businessinsider.com/best-parental-leave-policies-from-large-us-companies-2019-6#juniper-networks-employees-get-16-weeks-3
Breastfeeding and lactation policy	NYC model lactation accommodation policy https://www1.nyc.gov/site/cchr/law/lactation.page
Policy for sick leave and elderly care	The Hamilton project https://www.brookings.edu/wp-content/uploads/2017/10/es_10192017_expanding_access_earned_sick_leavemaestas.pdf

References

1. Kotter J. Change management. 1995. https://hbr.org/1995/05/leading-change-why-transformation-efforts-fail-2. Accessed on 10/6/2021.
2. Spector ND, Asante PA, Marcelin JR, et al. Women in pediatrics: progress, barriers, and opportunities for equity, diversity, and inclusion. Pediatrics. 2019;144(5):e20192149.
3. Silver JK, Ghalib R, Poorman JA, et al. (2008–2017) analysis of gender equity in leadership of physician-focused medical specialty societies. JAMA Intern Med. 2019;179(3):433–5.
4. Paturel A.. Where are all the women deans? (2021) Available at: https://www.aamc.org/news-insights/where-are-all-women-deans. Accessed June 6, 2021.
5. Murphy M, Callander JK, Dohan D, Grandis JR. Women's experiences of promotion and tenure in academic medicine and potential implications for gender disparities in career advancement: a qualitative analysis. JAMA Netw Open. 2021;4(9):e2125843. https://doi.org/10.1001/jamanetworkopen.2021.25843.
6. Richter KP, Clark L, Wick JA, Cruvinel E, Durham D, Shaw P, Shih GH, Befort CA, Simari RD. Women physicians and promotion in academic medicine. N Engl J Med. 2020;383(22):2148–57. https://doi.org/10.1056/NEJMsa1916935.
7. Silver JK, Poorman JA, Reilly JM, Spector ND, Goldstein R, Zafonte RD. Assessment of women physicians among authors of perspective-type articles published in high-impact Pediatric journals. JAMA Netw Open. 2018;1(3):e180802. https://doi.org/10.1001/jamanetworkopen.2018.0802.
8. Jagsi R, Means O, Lautenberger D, Jones RD, Griffith KA, Flotte TR, Gordon LK, Rexrode KM, Wagner LW, Chatterjee A. Women's representation among members and leaders of National Medical Specialty Societies. Acad Med. 2020;95(7):1043–9. https://doi.org/10.1097/ACM.0000000000003038.
9. Association of American Medical Colleges. Table 2.2. (2019) Number and percentage of ACGME residents and fellows by sex and specialty, 2017. 2018. Available at: https://www.aamc.org/data/workforce/reports/492576/2-2-chart.html. Accessed March 25, 2019.
10. Association of American Medical Colleges. Table 13 (2017): U.S. medical school faculty by sex, rank, and department, 2017. Available at: https://www.aamc.org/download/486102/data/17table13.pdf. Accessed January 10, 2019.
11. Association of American Medical Colleges. (2018) physician specialty data report: table 1.3. Number and percentage of active physicians by sex and specialty, 2017. Available at: https://www.aamc.org/data/workforce/reports/492560/1-3-chart.html. Accessed January 10, 2019.
12. Association of American Medical Colleges. Trends: U.S. medical school dean trends by dean type and sex, December 31 snapshots. 2019. Available at: https://www.aamc.org/download/495120/data/usmsf-trends-deans.xlsx. Accessed May 31, 2019.
13. Association of American Medical Colleges. Table C. Departmental chairs by department, sex, and race/ethnicity. 2018. Available at: https://www.aamc.org/download/495102/data/.
14. Johnson TJ, Ellison AM, Dalembert G, et al. Implicit bias in pediatric academic medicine. J Natl Med Assoc. 2017;109(3):156–63.
15. Kelly EH, Miskimen T, Rivera F, Peterson LE, Hingle ST. Women's wellness through equity and leadership (WEL): a program evaluation. Pediatrics. 2021;148(s2):e2021051440I.
16. Xierali IM, Nivet MA. The racial and ethnic composition and distribution of primary care physicians. J Health Care Poor Underserved. 2018;29(1):556–70.
17. Greenwood BN, Hardeman RR, Huang L, Sojourner A. Physician-patient racial concordance and disparities in birthing mortality for newborns. Proc Natl Acad Sci USA. 2020;117(35):21194–200.
18. Langley GJ, Moen RD, Nolan KM, et al. The improvement guide: a practical approach to enhancing organizational performance. 2nd ed. San Francisco: Jossey Bass; 2009.
19. Joshi M, Ransom E, Nash D, Ransom S. The healthcare quality book: vision, strategy, and tools. Chicago: Health Administration Press; 2014.
20. Zheng W, Kark R, Meister A. How women manage the gendered norms of leadership. Harv Bus Rev. 2018; https://hbr.org/2018/11/how-women-manage-the-gendered-norms-of-leadership. Last accessed on 10/14/2021

Chapter 10
Allies in Gender Equity Efforts in Pediatrics

Jorge F. Ganem, Glenn Rosenbluth, and Howard Yee Liu

Introduction

Gender inequities are pervasive and long-standing in medicine. The field of pediatrics is not exempt. The root causes of gender inequity and its harmful impacts on all aspects of our profession are described in detail throughout this book. In this chapter, we will focus on the role men have in creating and perpetuating gender inequities in medicine and specifically in pediatrics. We will also address the responsibilities men have in recognizing and eliminating gender inequity, from our day-to-day interactions in the workplace and beyond to broader systemic interventions. Some readers may ask, why should men have a voice in gender equity efforts? And more specifically, why should men write a chapter in a textbook dedicated to Women in Pediatrics? In an article describing the existing gender inequities in the field of cardiothoracic surgery which is dominated by men, Wood correctly calls out men as having an outsized responsibility to address gender disparities while proposing a set of principles for allies who are men to follow [34]. As men, we embrace our role as allies in promoting gender equity with purpose and humility. We write this chapter not proclaiming to be experts, but as partners who seek a deeper understanding of the problems and solutions. In the article titled "The coin model of privilege and critical allyship: implications for health," Nixon describes systems of inequity as

J. F. Ganem
PeaceHealth, Abigail Ln Eugene, OR, USA

G. Rosenbluth (✉)
University of California, San Francisco, San Francisco, CA, USA
e-mail: Glenn.Rosenbluth@ucsf.edu

H. Y. Liu
UNMC Department Psychiatry, UNMC COM, Nebraska Medical Center, Omaha, NE, USA
e-mail: hyliu@unmc.edu

N. D. Spector et al. (eds.), *Women in Pediatrics*,
https://doi.org/10.1007/978-3-030-98222-5_10

coins, with one side of the coin representing privilege and the other side representing oppression [20]. In our society and in medicine, women are the disadvantaged group when compared to men. As men, we recognize the inherent position of privilege we hold in our society and in our profession and how that privilege has served to create and maintain an unfair system which provides us multiple unearned advantages and benefits. As members of this privileged group, men should recognize that our experiences are different than those of women in our profession and that listening to women and believing them is critical our ability to understand the problem and engage in actionable change. We acknowledge that the burden of working toward dismantling oppressive systems does not lie with the oppressed and disadvantaged group. The work of men, as allies from an advantaged group, should be intentional, and it should focus not on correcting perceived flaws in women so they can succeed in inequitable systems. Working toward and achieving gender equity should not be viewed as a zero-sum game aiming to lift up women at the expense of men, but the goals of allyship should instead be directed to break down the unjust systems. As Nixon explains regarding solutions to inequity in the coin model, "The goal is not to move people from the bottom of the coin to the top, because both positions are unfair. Rather, the goal is to dismantle the systems (i.e., coins) causing the inequities" [20].

Defining Allyship

What does it mean to be an ally for gender equity and for women in healthcare? This is an essential question we must ask ourselves as we aspire to do the work of dismantling gender-based disparities in healthcare and beyond. In considering this question, Jain and colleagues emphasize that men should take deliberate action, that they should "walk the talk" [13]. How do we take deliberate action? It is important to first recognize that the journey toward allyship is dynamic and that allies and potential allies are often found along a continuum in terms of their readiness and ability to join the fray. Through this lens, we propose a practical and wide-ranging, although admittedly incomplete, definition of allyship composed of three main categories: listeners, amplifiers, and champions.

Listeners

Allyship has to start somewhere, and for some, being a listener can be the beginning of their allyship journey. Listeners give space and attention to the voices of those who are oppressed or disadvantaged. A listener may be someone who shows interest and wants to learn about gender equity but may not yet be ready to leap into a more active allyship role. Men can become allies through a commitment to learning about gender inequity, by listening to the experiences of women they work with, by attending presentations and workshops on gender equity and gender-based disparities, and through self-directed review of peer-reviewed literature and lay literature by thought leaders in the areas. During group meetings and professional conferences, men can be allies through active listening to the ideas and contributions of their women colleagues. Importantly, men can be active listeners by not interrupting women. Leaders can support listener allyship through intentional expectation-setting in group meetings and conferences including explicit rules and behavior norms for equitable and inclusive participation from all members of the group while avoiding practices favoring contributions from one gender over the other whether those meetings are in-person or virtual [9]. Listener allies can be vital in creating spaces that allow psychological safety for gender equity work to occur from the point of view of women [28]. Psychological safety is created within an environment that allows a person to feel included, safe to learn, safe to contribute, and safe to challenge the status quo, and with no fear of repercussions.

Another important aspect of listener allies is their potential to influence others to emulate similar allyship behavior through role modeling. It is plausible to suggest that men would be more likely to become active listeners and allies themselves if they observe other men such as their colleagues, particularly those they see as role models, step into the space, and take part in listener allyship behaviors such as participating in gender equity trainings or attending work meetings about important gender equity policies such as pay equity and parental leave.

Amplifiers

Amplifiers are allies who promote equity by using their position of privilege to magnify the voices of those who are minoritized or have less relative power. An example of how men can be amplifier allies is through professional sponsorship. Sponsorship is necessary for successful professional advancement. Men often wield large spheres of power and privilege within academic or professional organizations. In their study on mentorship and sponsorship, Patton and colleagues compare the differences women experience in professional advancement when they are mentored by men and find that women with sponsors who were men were offered professional advancement opportunities more often than women who were only mentored by men [23]. When allies who are men are able to extend their network of influence for the benefit of women colleagues, it can be crucial for their professional advancement. Men can amplify the work of women through timely sponsorship that is focused on promoting women to positions of leadership and power [4]. Men can also be amplifiers through dissemination of the message by ensuring gender equity is given a platform in important meetings and discussions.

Champions

Champion allies are those who are actively working to end gender inequity. Champions stand up and confront sexist behaviors in the workplace. Allies who are men can be champions by partnering with women and taking on the responsibility for creating policy, curricula, and trainings which address gender disparities within the organization and enacting systems change in compensation, leadership structure, and succession planning. Champions can make a difference not only through their actions but through the expectations they set for themselves and for other men in the organization. There is evidence that allyship behavior among individuals increases when they observe others confronting sexism· [4].

Awareness of Risks and Vulnerability

Allies can face backlash for their actions. Men may suffer penalties for rejecting stereotypical gendered norms that benefit them and may be looked upon as less competent by both men and women [6]. Men may also face criticism from the women they are allying with [14], and women may perceive an ally's actions as performative or may be skeptical of their intentions. Allies who are men can also risk jeopardizing women's action plans or proposals. "When aspiring male allies fail to understand the critical importance of partnering and collaborating with humility, there is a real risk that they may ultimately undermine women's initiatives by attempting to dominate them" [14].

How Men Contribute to Gender Inequity

In order to become key allies for gender equity, it is important for men to recognize the attitudes, beliefs, and actions responsible for creating, promoting, and maintaining inequitable systems. More importantly, it is crucial for men to acknowledge the substantial role we play in creating unequal and unsafe work environments for women through our perpetuation of stereotypes, biases, and systemic barriers to change.

Implicit bias is often defined as unconscious attitudes held by individuals about other individuals or groups. Everyone has implicit bias and while it may be difficult to eliminate, there may be ways to mitigate it. Examples of biases attributing negative qualities to women are numerous and are encountered frequently in medicine. They include beliefs that men are more capable leaders than women or that women should conform to specific roles in the workplace and in the home. A common instance of implicit gender bias is when women exhibit traits that are stereotypically associated with men, they are often labeled as "bossy" or "loud" or "aggressive," when men are often admired or rewarded for such behavior. Men contribute to gender inequities through the acceptance and amplification of these biases. Men are often in positions of power and are responsible for making individual and policy decisions about hiring, promotion, and compensation. Implicit bias influences men to make decisions in favor of other men and to the detriment of women. Active expressions of bias which contribute to gender inequity in the workplace are microaggressions. Periyakoil and colleagues describe microaggressions as actions and behaviors which can be subtle, verbal or nonverbal, and may arise from our implicit or explicit biases [24]. Biased comments and actions which may seem innocuous or harmless to men are often derogatory and injurious to women and contribute to eroding the psychological safety of the workplace. In their study, Periyakoil and colleagues found that women experience and report microaggressions in the workplace frequently, while men in the same workplaces are less likely to recognize that these microaggressions take place. In order to promote a more equitable workplace for everyone, men should confront these implicit gender biases and microaggressions, recognize them, challenge them, and work to eliminate them.

An even more blatant form of gender discrimination and bias is sexual harassment. Cross-sectional analyses of faculty and resident physicians have shown that sexual harassment is pervasive in medicine and contributes to unsafe working environments and lack of psychological safety. Sexual harassment and gender bias are primary reasons women leave the field of medicine [3, 16]. Men are not only responsible for creating and fostering a hostile workplace through active harassment, but they are also just as responsible when they are bystanders. When men ignore or tolerate sexual harassment, they send a clear message that women are not welcome in the workplace as peers and equals. A nourishing and psychologically safe work environment where everyone is given the opportunity to grow and thrive and women are treated equitably requires that men categorically and actively denounce sexual harassment in policy and day-to-day interactions.

It is important for men to recognize that gender bias and inequities are compounded when the victim of these transgressions belongs to or identifies as a member of another marginalized group in medicine and society. The term intersectionality initially was used to describe situations unique to Black women when compared to white women or Black men. The definition of intersectionality has expanded to include other instances where, as an example, one individual may be the victim of gender bias and racial bias at the same time and how that experience differs from individuals experiencing only one of those biases.

Another important factor to consider is how men contribute to gender inequity through building and sustaining systems that are inherently unequal. Leadership structures in medicine are often set up to propagate gender inequity through lack of transparent succession plans. Traditional medicine promotion structures facilitate gender inequity through the advancement of candidates who are similar in gender and ethnicity, (i.e., white men). Lack of defined term limits for high-level leadership positions also create disparities through promotion of a patriarchal structure without allowing opportunity for women or other underrepresented groups to gain power. Studies show that women benefit from men as sponsors in order to achieve positions in leadership for which they are similarly qualified or more highly qualified for than men. The failure of men in leadership positions to recognize the opportunity to sponsor well-qualified women for leadership opportunities is a major driver of gender inequity.

The Case for Gender Equity

Internal Motivation for Gender Equity

As alluded to above, many men default to concerns that we exist in a zero-sum system regarding gender equity. This zero-sum model can be viewed analogous to a seesaw – in order to elevate one side of the seesaw, the other group must naturally be lowered. However, this model ignores an underlying evidence base which demonstrates that by lifting one group, both can achieve more. Put another way, creating space for women and others who have been historically marginalized doesn't necessarily consume space – rather the process has the potential to create more space for everyone.

Meaningful allyship, sponsorship, and other direct support often require us to reassess existing frameworks (see Chap. 12). For example, when describing or defining leadership traits, we often use different language to describe leaders who are men based on specific traits [27]. These traits may lead us to identify and hire leaders with leadership styles that are traditionally associated with men (e.g., top-down/autocratic leadership styles) which may or may not be well-suited to particular work environments. (It's important to acknowledge that existing biases may lead us to view these same traits less positively when they apply to women.) Lack of attention to gender-based perceptions leaves us vulnerable to hiring leaders with gaps in their skills sets related to emotional intelligence, more democratic approaches, and focus on inspiring and transforming individuals – traits which have become increasingly more important as our healthcare workforce continues to diversify.

There continue to be gender-based differences in perceptions of bosses and leaders – specifically that both genders tend to favor having a male boss [19]. This is likely multifactorial, but it is hard to ignore the ingrained stereotypes about what makes a "good leader." Linda Kaboolian writes about the challenge that leadership within healthcare has been mostly defined by examples of men and how this can "lessen the chances that women will be promoted into these coveted positions" [7]. As individuals rise through systems, they are more likely to have seen men in leadership roles, and also women leaders may be more likely to be impacted by stereotype threats. The burden must fall on allies who are men to help call out these stereotypes and create greater equity in leadership roles.

Inequity and lack of diversity in the workplace hurt everyone. There is a large body of data associating diversity with improved organizational outcomes. Women in leadership roles may be more likely to coach and mentor junior faculty which benefits all by creating a stronger organizational pipeline [7]. Diversity in organizational leadership has been associated with improved organizational performance. A report by McKinsey found that companies in the top quartile for gender diversity on executive teams were consistently more likely to have above-average profitability – as much as 50% higher share performance – when women are well-represented in leadership [10]. However, this same study reported that more than half of companies have made "little or no progress, and some have even gone backward" with respect to diversity in their leadership teams. This is a reminder that there is much work to do, and men must be allies and accomplices in this work. As long as men remain disproportionately overrepresented in leadership, they continue to hold the power to change the system.

Specifically, in healthcare, women in leadership roles may help healthcare organizations grow more effectively than they would with men in those roles. For example, women may be more likely to promote family-friendly policies. These policies benefit all by making it less likely that individuals will leave their organization – turnover which the Association of American Medical Colleges (AAMC) estimates at $250,000 to almost $1 million per physician. In a time when more men are taking advantage of family leave policies and taking on larger roles in child-rearing, these policies may have substantial impact on supporting the workforce [21].

Beyond "profit motivation" or "bottom line," there are some very practical and likely more compelling reasons to promote gender equity within healthcare. Perhaps the most basic and practical is improved mortality for our patients. We have data that men and women practice differently, and in fact these differences may lead to the result that patients cared for by women may have improved outcomes [30]. This difference has been seen more specifically in surgical populations, in which patients cared for by female surgeons may have decreased mortality [33]. In patients suffering from heart attacks, having a female provider actually eliminated a well-documented disparity: rather than decreased survival in female patients, when the treating physician was female, men and women had equivalent outcomes.

These reported differences in survival may be due to many factors – likely some combination of the fact that women are more likely to follow established clinical guidelines and provide more patient-centered communication and more psychosocial counseling. An interesting proposition in the surgical report by Wallis et al. is that there may be greater openness to collaboration, "which might avert scenarios that could otherwise result in the 'failure to rescue' phenomenon" [33].

Finally, in the realm of academic pediatrics, we must acknowledge historical and current disparities resulting in disproportionately fewer women in medical research – both as researchers and as subjects. Women represent a smaller share of authors on published research than men – and though this disparity is improving, women still represent less than 50% of authors and are substantially less likely to be in the senior author position [11]. This, together with the fact that men and women are likely to focus on different areas of research, suggests that we may face significant gaps in the medical literature which can be closed if more women are supported doing research.

Women have also been historically underrepresented as subjects in clinical trials. Beyond the ethical disparity this creates, there is also a financial cost resulting from delayed identification of side effects which may affect half of the population. The US General Accounting Office reported that over the years from 1997 to 2000, eight of ten drugs removed from the US market were removed due to side effects which occurred disproportionately, or exclusively, in women [22]. While we could not find specific evidence that women are more likely to include women in their clinical trials, and the FDA currently requires that women and minorities be included in government-funded clinical trials, we feel comfortable postulating that increasing the number of clinical trials overseen by women could potentially decrease disparities in outcomes.

Men as Allies in the Workplace

Women make up 36.3% of the physician workforce in the USA and 64.3% of active pediatricians [1]. They are 60% of faculty in departments in pediatrics yet only 31% of the chairs of these departments [2]. As we consider allyship in a workplace that boasts a substantial presence of women, we must address both structural and individual factors [5].

On the structural side, leaders who are men must pay attention to the policies which drive equity and the culture which bolsters or undermines these policies. This includes workplace flexibility, workforce and talent development, pay parity and transparency in the organization, and the creation of a safe environment and consequences related to sexual harassment and gender bias. On the individual side, it is imperative that allies progress along the continuum from listener to amplifier to champion as outlined earlier. Examples are outlined in Table 10.1.

Regarding structural allyship, here are four domains that every leader should address at their workplace:

Workplace Flexibility The trend toward flexible workplaces began years ago but has accelerated markedly in the COVID-19 pandemic as many individuals have

Table 10.1 Five case scenarios of allyship

Scenario	Listeners	Amplifiers	Champions
Academic: A mid-career woman colleague is seeking promotion to associate professor, but the leadership roles in the department are predominantly filled by men with little turnover	You listen to the concerns of your colleague	You elevate this concern to the chair, vice chair, or division director with the permission of the woman colleague	You use your leverage as a leader or you advocate with the appropriate leader(s) to create succession planning and an inclusive search process for leadership roles at all levels. You challenge the professors and senior faculty to sponsor women and BIPOC candidates for leadership roles both within and outside of the department

Table 10.1 (continued)

Scenario	Listeners	Amplifiers	Champions
Administrative: An early career woman pediatrician compares notes with a male colleague and discovers that she was offered 10% less on her starting salary	You actively listen to your colleague and commiserate with the unfairness of the situation	With the permission of your colleague who is a woman, you bring this pay discrepancy up with your immediate supervisor	You are continuously campaigning for gender pay equity and transparent pay practices at your workplace. If you are in a leadership role, you have worked with your DEI leadership to ensure pay parity is monitored and corrected
Clinical: A patient addresses the PGY-3 woman physician by first name during rounds but addresses the male intern as "doctor"	After rounds, you listen attentively to your female colleague as she states how commonly this occurs	During rounds, you speak up in the moment to correct the patient and address your colleague as "Dr. X"	You speak up in the moment and bring this example as an agenda item to the monthly faculty meeting and graduate medical education team. You highlight that this behavior occurs frequently and that it is the attending physician's role to address the behavior immediately. You work with your leadership team to arrange bystander training for attendings and trainees
Culture: The required department meeting is scheduled at 5 p.m. on a weekday. This conflicts with childcare responsibilities for many young parents – especially women faculty	You solicit and listen to the concerns from women colleagues	You elevate these concerns to the next level so that department leadership is aware. You bring up the concept of face time bias to leaders	You advocate with the senior leadership team to poll the faculty on the best times for meetings. You reschedule the meetings that you chair to coincide with the recommendations of parents of young children.
Regulatory: a medical student confides that she was sexually harassed by a male chief resident in the program.	You listen and report this concern to your title IX coordinator	You listen and report this concern to the title IX coordinator. You offer to bring this up to the GME, student affairs and faculty affairs leadership teams, if the student gives permission	You listen and report this concern to your title IX coordinator. You ensure that sexual harassment training is more than a "check box" compliance module, but a regular theme to be discussed via grand rounds, interview preparation, etc. you follow through with your leadership team to ensure that confirmed perpetrators are disciplined

been working from home or working hybrid schedules. Women are facing amplified work-life conflict due to the gendered expectation that women will remain the primary caretaker for families – both children and aging parents or relatives. As COVID-19 disrupted schools and childcare providers and created acute and chronic care needs for loved ones, it has placed tremendous and disproportionate strain on women [18]. The role of allies is to organize listening sessions for women in the workplace and to advocate for policies to support flexibility in caregiving roles. This could take the form of direct financial support for women and their families, investing in childcare infrastructure, and implementing family supportive policies. Practically, this could mean moving meeting times to avoid drop-off/pickup times for parents of school-age children. However, policies alone are not enough to change culture. One study of biomedical faculty showed a significant gap between utilization and expressed need for workplace flexibility: 33.4% of women faculty reported using the benefits available to them, while 44.4% of women reported wanting to use them [25]. A "culture of overwork" was cited as a significant barrier to fully utilizing workplace flexibility benefits due to the inexorable push for publications, clinical productivity, etc. In other words, allies must not rest when an inclusive policy is passed. They must anticipate cultural barriers and address them to ensure that women are not penalized for utilizing flextime policies.

Workforce and Talent Development In many academic health centers, significant attention is paid to the diversity of the pipeline at the front end: medical students, residents, and early career faculty. However, relatively less attention is paid to talent development for women in their mid-career who aspire to assume senior leadership roles as evidenced by the ongoing gap in promotion to professor and the gender disparities in senior academic leadership roles such as chair or dean. One simple measure of the health of the pipeline is to ask every leader who is a man in a senior leadership team, "How many women are you personally sponsoring or mentoring? How many of them identify as underrepresented in medicine? How many are mid-career?" From training search committees in inclusive practices to nominating women for awards and leadership roles to creating term limits for succession planning, allies must be proactive in workforce development. Allies can also nurture talent development by supporting executive coaching for women at all career phases.

Pay Equity and Transparency Reams of data have demonstrated that women in medicine continue to face disparities in equitable pay. Most of the gender pay gap literature continues to be generated by women and is often unfunded [17]. For example, one analysis of 39 physician compensation studies reported no funding or no relevant funding in 59% of those studies. Allies can take tangible steps to achieve gender pay parity in departments and in organizations by speaking up about existing gender pay gaps, employing transparent methodologies to close the gaps, and funding ongoing research and consultation on gender pay gaps. The onus for change lies primarily with senior leaders including chairs and deans of academic health centers and HR and C-suite members of hospital leadership teams. Structured compensation may be one path toward creating transparent pay steps and increments for women, but true pay equity will require a concerted approach to increasing the representation of women in the most highly compensated specialties and senior leadership roles [12]. Equitable pay for women physicians may aid in overall resilience as there is emerging data that debt burden increases burnout for women physicians [31].

Workplace Safety and Sexual Harassment Decades of data underscore that sexual harassment of women continues to be a persistent, pervasive problem for women at all levels of healthcare and academia [8]. As Paula A. Johnson and Sheila Widnall, Co-Chairs of the Committee on the Impacts of Sexual Harassment in Academia for the National Academies of Sciences, Engineering, and Medicine (NASEM) state: "*We are encouraged by the research that suggests that the most potent predictor of sexual harassment is organizational climate – the degree to which those in the organization perceive that sexual harassment is or is not tolerated.*" Allies must do more than direct women colleagues and trainees to the Title IX Coordinator if an infraction occurs. Allies must also take steps to address culture by speaking up about the need for psychological safety at work and supporting infrastructure to create an inclusive environment. This includes being proactive to support climate surveys, engaging in training programs that target behavior, encouraging leaders to speak up about behavioral expectations both at work and in work-related settings such as conferences, and specifying consequences when those expectations are violated. Ultimately, the goal should be to create a culture of transparency and accountability regarding sexual harassment and workplace safety.

Men as Allies outside the Workplace

Men have a large role to play in gender equity outside the workplace as well. While not all professional women are in domestic relationships with partners who are men, a very common scenario in our society is for professional women to be married to or partnered with a man who also has professional duties outside the home. In this section, we will focus on allyship by men in these relationship structures. Household inequities between working partners have a significantly detrimental impact on the career arc of women physicians. A study by Starmer and colleagues examining factors associated with the division of household responsibilities for pediatricians in the early or middle of their career demonstrated existing inequities between men and women in domestic relationships including the findings that pediatricians who were men spent less time on concrete household tasks than women, and that women were more likely to carry the primary responsibility of completing most household tasks [29]. Jones and colleagues describe how the COVID-19 pandemic has not only contributed to exacerbating gender inequities in the workplace but has also served to further shift the already existing imbalance of home responsibilities toward women due to school closures and childcare disruptions [15]. A recent study examining the experiences of men and women in spousal relationships as they negotiated time and space working from home during the COVID-19 pandemic showed that men's workspace and time for work at home were more defined with clear boundaries than that of women, who often had to spread their worktime throughout the day and were required to find workspace throughout the home [32]. In their article "Gender Equity Starts in the Home," Smith and Johnson assert that equity in domestic partnerships can promote gender equity by increasing the potential for women to be more productive and successful at work [26]. This argument proposes that equal partnerships at home provide both partners the opportunity to be flexible in finding balance between responsibilities at work and at home without the need for one partner to sacrifice career growth and development at the expense of the other.

Conclusion

Gender inequity hurts everyone; it is not a problem affecting only women. The field of pediatrics is not exempt from gender inequity despite being a specialty where the majority of physicians are women. Men have an outsized role to play in the elimination of gender inequities through meaningful allyship in the workplace and as equal partners outside the workplace. The case for gender equity is clear on an individual and an organizational level. Achieving gender equity is not a zero-sum game; everyone benefits from more diverse and equitable work environments. As members of a privileged group, men should take responsibility and work to enact change in their day-to-day interactions, as allies, sponsors, and mentors, and as advocates for policy and systems change.

References

1. 2020 Physician Specialty Data Report Executive Summary. n.d. AAMC. Retrieved December 30, 2021, from https://www.aamc.org/data-reports/data/2020-physician-specialty-data-report-executive-summary.
2. 2020 U.S. Medical School Faculty. n.d. AAMC. Retrieved December 30, 2021, from https://www.aamc.org/data-reports/faculty-institutions/interactive-data/2020-us-medical-school-faculty
3. Arnold LF, Zargham SR, Gordon CE, McKinley WI, Bruenderman EH, Weaver JL, Benns MV, Egger ME, Motameni AT. Sexual harassment during residency training: a cross-sectional analysis. Am Surg. 2020;86(1):65–72.
4. Ayyala MS, Skarupski K, Bodurtha JN, González-Fernández M, Ishii LE, Fivush B, Levine RB. Mentorship is not enough: exploring sponsorship and its role in career advancement in academic medicine. Acad Med. 2019;94(1):94–100. https://doi.org/10.1097/ACM.0000000000002398.
5. Bilal M, Balzora S, Pochapin MB, Oxentenko AS. The need for Allyship in achieving gender equity in gastroenterology. Am J Gastroenterol. 2021; Publish Ahead of Print. https://doi.org/10.14309/ajg.0000000000001508.
6. Bosak J, Kulich C, Rudman L, Kinahan M. Be an advocate for others, unless you are a man: backlash against gender-atypical male job candidates. Psychol Men Masculinity. 2018;19(1):156–65.
7. Chamorro-Premuzic T, Gallop C. 7 Leadership Lessons Men Can Learn from Women. Harvard Business Review. 2020, April 1. https://hbr.org/2020/04/7-leadership-lessons-men-can-learn-from-women.
8. Committee on the Impacts of Sexual Harassment in Academia, Committee on Women in Science, Engineering, and Medicine, Policy and Global Affairs, & National Academies of Sciences, Engineering, and Medicine. In: Johnson PA, Widnall SE, Benya FF, editors. Sexual

harassment of women: climate, culture, and consequences in academic sciences, engineering, and medicine. National Academies Press; 2018. https://doi.org/10.17226/24994.

9. Dhawan N, Carnes M, Byars-Winston A, Duma N. Videoconferencing etiquette: promoting gender equity during virtual meetings. J Women's Health. 2021;30(4):460–5. https://doi.org/10.1089/jwh.2020.8881.
10. Dixon-Fyle S, Dolan K, Hunt V, Prince S. n.d. Diversity wins: how inclusion matters. McKinsey & Company. Retrieved December 30, 2021, from https://www.mckinsey.com/featured-insights/diversity-and-inclusion/diversity-wins-how-inclusion-matters.
11. Gayet-Ageron A, Poncet A, Perneger T. Comparison of the contributions of female and male authors to medical research in 2000 and 2015: a cross-sectional study. BMJ Open. 2019;9(2):e024436. https://doi.org/10.1136/bmjopen-2018-024436.
12. Hayes SN, Noseworthy JH, Farrugia G. A structured compensation plan results in equitable physician compensation. Mayo Clin Proc. 2020;95(1):35–43. https://doi.org/10.1016/j.mayocp.2019.09.022.
13. Jain S, Madani K, Flint L, Swaroop M, Liu H, Varghese T, Sinha M, Silver J. What does it mean to be a male ally? Implementing meaningful change in gender representation in medicine. J Am Coll Surg. 2020;230(3):355–6. https://doi.org/10.1016/j.jamcollsurg.2019.12.001.
14. Johnson WB, Smith DG. How men can become better allies to women. Harvard Business Review. 2018, October 12. https://hbr.org/2018/10/how-men-can-become-better-allies-to-women.
15. Jones Y, Durand V, Morton K, Ottolini M, Shaughnessy E, Spector ND, O'Toole J. Collateral damage: how COVID-19 is adversely impacting women physicians. J Hosp Med. 2020;15(8):507–9. https://doi.org/10.12788/jhm.3470
16. Komaromy M, Bindman AB, Haber RJ, Sande MA. Sexual harassment in medical training. N Engl J Med. 1993;328(5):322–6. https://doi.org/10.1056/NEJM199302043280507.
17. Larson AR, Cawcutt KA, Englander MJ, Pitt SC, Ansari E, Liu HY, Silver JK. Representation of women in authorship and dissemination of analyses of physician compensation. JAMA Netw Open. 2020;3(3):e201330. https://doi.org/10.1001/jamanetworkopen.2020.1330.
18. National Academies of Sciences, E. Short-term strategies for addressing the impacts of the COVID-19 pandemic on women's workforce participation. 2021. https://doi.org/10.17226/26303.
19. Newport F, Wilke J. Americans Still Prefer a Male Boss. Gallup.Com. 2013, November 11. https://news.gallup.com/poll/165791/americans-prefer-male-boss.aspx.
20. Nixon SA. The coin model of privilege and critical allyship: implications for health. BMC Public Health. 2019;19(1):1637. https://doi.org/10.1186/s12889-019-7884-9.
21. Nutter DO, Bond JS, Coller BS, D'Alessandri RM, Gewertz BL, Nora LM, Perkins JP, Shomaker TS, Watson RT. Measuring faculty effort and contributions in medical education. Acad Med. 2000;75(2):200–7. https://doi.org/10.1097/00001888-200002000-00025.
22. Office, U. S. G. A. Drug safety: most drugs withdrawn in recent years had greater health risks for women. n.d. Retrieved December 30, 2021, from https://www.gao.gov/products/gao-01-286r.
23. Patton EW, Griffith KA, Jones RD, Stewart A, Ubel PA, Jagsi R. Differences in mentor-mentee sponsorship in male vs female recipients of National Institutes of Health Grants. JAMA Intern Med. 2017;177(4):580. https://doi.org/10.1001/jamainternmed.2016.9391.
24. Periyakoil VS, Chaudron L, Hill EV, Pellegrini V, Neri E, Kraemer HC. Common types of gender-based microaggressions in medicine. Acad Med. 2020;95(3):450–7. https://doi.org/10.1097/ACM.0000000000003057.
25. Shauman K, Howell LP, Paterniti DA, Beckett LA, Villablanca AC. Barriers to career flexibility in academic medicine: A qualitative analysis of reasons for the underutilization of family-friendly policies, and implications for institutional change and department chair leadership. Acad Med. 2018;93(2):246–55. https://doi.org/10.1097/ACM.0000000000001877.
26. Smith DG, Johnson WB. Gender Equity Starts in the Home. Harvard Business Review. 2020, May 4. https://hbr.org/2020/05/gender-equity-starts-in-the-home.

27. Smith DG, Rosenstein JE, Nikolov MC. The different words we use to describe male and female leaders. Harvard Business Review. 2018, May 25. https://hbr.org/2018/05/the-different-words-we-use-to-describe-male-and-female-leaders.
28. Sonnenberg LK, Do V, LeBlanc C, Busari JO. Six ways to get a grip by calling-out racism and enacting allyship in medical education. Can Med Educat J. 2021; https://doi.org/10.36834/cmej.71566.
29. Starmer AJ, Frintner MP, Matos K, Somberg C, Freed G, Byrne BJ. Gender discrepancies related to Pediatrician work-life balance and household responsibilities. Pediatrics. 2019;144(4):e20182926. https://doi.org/10.1542/peds.2018-2926.
30. Tsugawa Y, Jena A, Figueroa J, Orav E, Blumenthal D, JHA, A. Comparison of hospital mortality and readmission rates for Medicare patients treated by male vs female physicians. JAMA Intern Med. 2017;177:206–13. https://doi.org/10.1001/jamainternmed.2016.7875.
31. Verduzco-Gutierrez M, Larson AR, Capizzi AN, Bean AC, Zafonte RD, Odonkor CA, Bosques G, Silver JK. How physician compensation and education debt affects financial stress and burnout: a survey study of women in physical medicine and rehabilitation. PM&R. 2021;13(8):836–44. https://doi.org/10.1002/pmrj.12534.
32. Waismel-Manor R, Wasserman V, Shamir-Balderman O. No room of her own: married couples' negotiation of workspace at home during COVID-19. Sex Roles. 2021;1–14 https://doi.org/10.1007/s11199-021-01246-1.
33. Wallis CJ, Ravi B, Coburn N, Nam RK, Detsky AS, Satkunasivam R. Comparison of post-operative outcomes among patients treated by male and female surgeons: a population based matched cohort study. BMJ. 2017;j4366 https://doi.org/10.1136/bmj.j4366.
34. Wood DE. How can men be good allies for women in surgery? #HeForShe. J Thorac Dis. 2021;13(1):492–501. https://doi.org/10.21037/jtd-2020-wts-11

Chapter 11
Research, Funding, and Publication for Women in Pediatrics

Karen M. Wilson and Beth A. Tarini

Introduction

Research is the gold standard by which academic success is measured. There is no higher achievement in medicine than the Nobel Prize; up until 2014, only 16 women have ever received a Nobel Prize for their contributions to research [1]; seven additional have been awarded since then. But Nobel Prize winners are cultivated, through long years of training, and then graduated experiences as faculty and independent observers. The physician-scientist pipeline, as it is called for those who have a medical degree and pursue research-focused career, provides an orderly series of steps, from residency, to fellowship, to career development awards, through larger independent grants (Fig. 11.1) [2]. However, there is a concept called the "leaky pipeline," [3] which describes the loss of diverse talent, particularly people from groups underrepresented in medicine and women, all along the physician-scientist pipeline. A study in the early 2000s found that there had been a steady decline in the percentage of women medical students who intended to pursue medical careers [4]; while we don't have current data to see the percentage of women medical students who are interested in or contemplating a research career, the challenges in obtaining research funding can't have helped.

K. M. Wilson (✉)
Department of Pediatrics and the Clinical and Translational Sciences Institute, University of Rochester School of Medicine, Rochester, NY, USA
e-mail: Karen_Wilson@urmc.rochester.edu

B. A. Tarini
Center for Translational Research, Children's National Research Institute, Children's National Hospital, The George Washington University, Society for Pediatric Research, Silver Spring, MD, USA
e-mail: btarini@childrensnational.org

N. D. Spector et al. (eds.), *Women in Pediatrics*,
https://doi.org/10.1007/978-3-030-98222-5_11

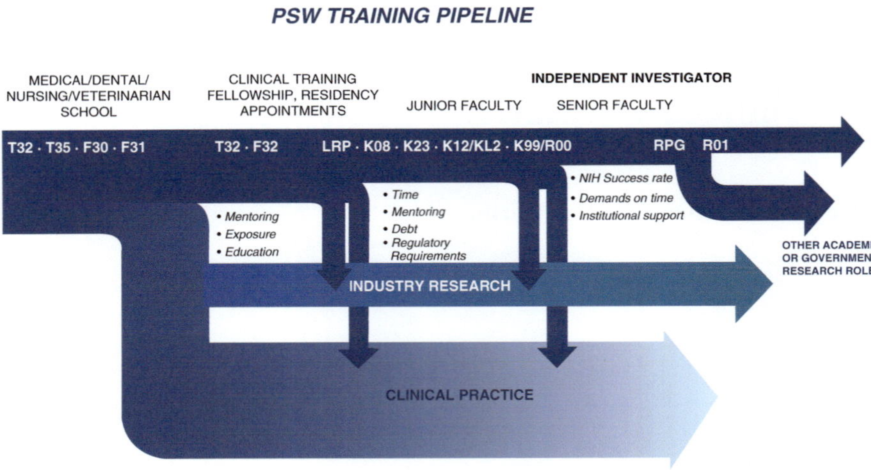

Fig. 11.1 NIH support for the physician-scientist pipeline https://acd.od.nih.gov/documents/reports/PSW_Report_ACD_06042014.pdf

Women have been vibrant contributors to medical research. Nobel Prizes in Physiology have gone to Gerty Cori, for her work on carbohydrate metabolism; Rosalyn Yalow, for developing the radioimmunoassay; and Dr. Francoise Barre-Sinoussi, for discovering the way that HIV is spread, among many others. Yet there have been other women scientists, such as Rosalind Franklin, whose critical contributions were undervalued or overlooked [5]. As a result, it is important to recognize as we discuss the role of women in pediatric research, that we don't forget about the persistent bias and additional challenges met by physicians of color, and from other underrepresented backgrounds. The leaky pipeline is just as leaky, and perhaps more so, for these groups.

Funding

Training researchers and conducting research require funding. For training medical researchers, the federal government funds numerous programs throughout the training pathway, from medical school through faculty (Fig. 11.1). Pediatric researcher trainees are eligible for most, if not all, of these programs. In 2001, 10% of all pediatric residency graduates pursued a career in research, far below that of other specialties such as internal medicine [6, 7]. Pediatric research at the NIH is funded across institutes, and efforts are being made to harmonize pediatric research activities across the NIH, including improving training for pediatric researchers of the next generation. One such trans-NIH initiative (NIH is made up of 27 institutes and centers) is NIH Pediatric Research Consortium (N-PeRC), which was established in 2018 [8]. Concerns have been raised that the current NIH training funding mechanisms have privileged existing training programs over new programs, thus limiting the ability to diversify the funding pool [9]. The current proportion of women who comprise pediatric research training programs is not available.

Foundation grants provide an important source of funding for pediatric research trainees, as well as established faculty. Foundation grants can range from a few thousand to a few hundred thousand dollars. These funding mechanisms are incredibly important and often undervalued by the broader academic community because of both their size and their low or absent indirect cost funding to institutions. Yet, these funding mechanisms provide critical funding to smaller scope research projects, which are common among pediatric trainees as well as established faculty who are working on new or emerging areas that may be seen as high risk by federal agencies.

The goal standard of research accomplishment is to receive an NIH award. For the junior faculty, that award is often a career development award. For a mid-level faculty member, that is often an R01 award. The challenge with this standard is that it excludes pediatric researchers who do not conduct research that aligns with the mission of the NIH. This could potentially exclude areas in which women pediatric researchers may focus.

While the largest group of funded investigators by the NIH is physicians with an MD only (51%), MD/PhDs are significantly overrepresented in NIH grant funding compared to their overall numbers. While there are many routes to an MD/PhD, the NIH funds the Medical Scientist Training Program (MSTP) at 43 institutions, which supports almost 1000 trainees each year. In 2011, women made up 39% of MD/PhD applicants, 37% of matriculants, and 42% of graduates [2]. However, a deeper dive into gender in MSTP programs in 2018 found that women were more likely to apply to programs that were lower in *U.S. News & World Report* ranking [10]. MSTP trainees are far more likely to receive their PhD in a biological or physical science, rather than social sciences, health services research, or clinical informatics [2]. Increasing opportunities for MD/PhD candidates to obtain their doctorate in a more clinical field is an opportunity to appeal to a broader audience, including potentially more women.

While we can see the overall funding patterns for physicians and physician scientists, it's more difficult to know how that is reflected within pediatrics. Since women make up a much larger share of graduating physicians, it should follow that they would have higher representation in grant funding. However, there are few data on whether this is the case. In fact, a study of a pediatric resident research grant program found that women asked for less money, and received lower scores than men, even controlling for advanced degrees (of which men had more) [11]. If these disparities are starting in training, they are likely to persist.

While the percentage of women MDs who are NIH research project grant holders has increased from 17% in the mid-1990s to 29% in 2014, this growth has actually been slower for MD/PhDs, who were also at 17% in the mid-1990s, and were at 22% in 2014 [2]. In 2012, the research project grant award rate was not different by gender, with men successful 23% of the time, and women successful 24% [2].

There are multiple reasons why women may be underrepresented in research grant awards. The physician-scientist pipeline is not forgiving; women who take time during residency or fellowship to care for children may find completing a project that may launch their career and stimulate their interest in research daunting, and mentors may dissuade them from taking this path. Academic careers are often less financially rewarding, and thus young women may pragmatically decide that a clinical career provides more security. Of course, these decisions are not only being made by women; it is likely that having a process that rewards and supports less traditional pathways and time off would also encourage more talented men to enter research careers. Alternatively, the system of K to R transitions has historically relied on sponsorship and mentorship, and we know that women often don't get the same opportunities to engage with more senior faculty as men.

Publications

From 2000 to 2015, women increased from 32% of authors to 41% of authors in the *Annals of Internal Medicine*, though in 2016 only 16% were senior authors [12]. The field of pediatrics provides an interesting case study in authorship representation by gender. Pediatrics is one of only two specialties in medicine where the proportion of practicing physicians who are women is over 50%. In 2017, women were 72% of pediatric residents, 63% of practicing physicians, and 57% of academic pediatricians [13]. Fishman et al. (2017) [14] assessed the prevalence of authorship by women in three high impact pediatrics journals from 2001 to 2016, as well as editorial board membership. The overall proportion of women first authors increased from 40% to 58% ($p < .001$); the proportion of senior authors increased from 29% to 38% ($P < .001$) [14]. They concluded that women first authors are underrepresented in comparison to women junior faculty, while women senior authors are represented in number similar to women senior faculty. A more recent study examined the representation of women authors in perspective articles in high impact pediatric journals. The proportion of women first authors was 42%, and this was even lower among the authors of articles in journals where the perspectives were considered "scholarly" (15–44%), compared to "narrative" (53% vs. 66%) [15].

This disparity is even more apparent in other fields. A review of cardiovascular clinical trials published in high impact journals found that only 9% of first authors and 10% of last authors were women, and this was even more striking in large and procedurally oriented trials [16]. More recently, the COVID-19 pandemic has highlighted discrepancies in the ability of women to balance the increased child care demands of at-home schooling with the demands of an academic career, and in fact a 2020 report found that women's shares of papers from 2019 to 2020 decreased by 14% for first author papers, 3% for senior author papers, and 5% for overall representation [17].

Women also lag in placement on editorial boards. The Fishman et al. (2017) article also assessed editorial board membership at the three high impact pediatric journals, and found that overall representation of women increased from 18% in 2001 to 40% in 2016 ($p < .001$).

As we look at the leaky pipeline to professor and leadership positions for women, we must recognize the role that research and scholarship play. Department chairs are often chosen for their research portfolios, rather than their management skills. Thus, fewer women choosing research careers will mean fewer being considered for these roles. There is certainly debate about whether physician-scientists make the best chairs, but to have gender equity in academic pediatrics, we must also consider the value of nonphysician scientists in leadership roles, and work to make research an attractive and viable option for women.

Training and Transition to Faculty

Fellowships

Most pediatric-focused fellowships involve a combination of clinical and research training. To complete training for many pediatric board specialties, individuals must engage in scholarly activity and produce a work product [18]. The options for activities vary, but research, grants, and published manuscripts are among them. There are research-focused fellowships available for pediatricians. One of the most well-known has been the Robert Wood Johnson Clinical Scholars Program (RWJ CSP) [19]. In recent years, this program has moved away from funding single MD development to funding team-based multidisciplinary model. A program run by alumnae of NCSP, National Clinician Scholars Program, has emerged to assume the mission of the original RWJ CSP [20].

In many cases, fellowship might be the first time that a trainee encounters the opportunity to lead a research project. Often fellowship is the time when a trainee has specific and substantial time set aside to spend focused time on research. Times vary by specific fellowship and across fellowship sites within a specialty. Admittedly, this time can be scheduled and "fit in" alongside other clinical duties like overnight calls, for example. This can create obvious challenges for women, who are often primary caregivers, with balancing workload and family responsibilities. The importance of mentorship to fellowship research success cannot be understated [21].

Early Faculty

Fellowship is also an important time in a physician researcher's career because it provides the foundation upon which a future faculty position is built [22]. Navigating the search and negotiation of a junior faculty position can be challenging for any trainee. Women face additional hurdles related to their socialized approach to negotiation, as well as the culture's reaction to their negotiation style [23]. It is critical that a faculty member who is committed to a physician-investigator career have the necessary administrative, capital, and mentorship resources to achieve their early career goals [24]. For example, start-up support, (i.e., institutional funds to provide for research-based activities such as faculty salary, research staff salary, non-personnel-related research costs) has been linked to increased success of NIH funding [25]. Unfortunately, studies outside of pediatrics have demonstrated that women faculty have been shown to be receive less institutional support, especially in the basic sciences [26]. The legacy of less institutional support for women researchers compounded with their caregiver roles has been shown to severely impact their productivity [27]. Similarly, flexible employment, including part time, for research intensive faculty is particularly relevant for women who may have the primary or majority role as caregiver in the home [29, 30].

Promotion

Progressing through the ranks of academic medicine can be a grind. While promotion is anchored in achievement in scholarship, the road can be fraught with challenges, both personal and professional, individual, and institutional. Physician-scientists Drs. Megan Moreno and Rachel Katzenellenbogen have encouraged women faculty to utilize the a socioecological (SEM) framework to plan and assess their career growth [28]. The SEM framework places the faculty member within larger contexts which include their mentors, colleagues, and teams, their academic environment, and their professional society. Within this framework, faculty can consider their academic achievement (e.g., publications, grants, etc.) as well as their support within and outside of their institution (e.g., mentorship, sponsorship, administrative and capital resources).

Research Leadership

After achieving success in leadership, some physician-investigators go on to leadership positions. Such leadership paths include dean positions (research, medical school), department chairs, vice chairs of research, or chief scientific/research officers of research institutes. However, as one moves through these ranks, the prevalence of women decreases [13]. Women's representation among pediatric research professional societies is slightly better [13]. While progress has been made in the support of women pediatric researchers, there is room for continued improvement [31].

References

1. Modgil S, Gill R, Lakshmi Sharma V, Velassery S, Anand A. Nobel nominations in science: constraints of the fairer sex. Ann Neurosci. 2018;25(2):63–79. https://doi.org/10.1159/000481906.
2. National Institutes of Health. Physician-Scientist Workforce Working Group Report; 2014.
3. Goulden M, Mason MA, Frasch K. Keeping women in the science pipeline. Ann Am Acad Pol Soc Sci. 2011;638(1):141–62. https://doi.org/10.1177/0002716211416925.
4. Guelich JM, Singer BH, Castro MC, Rosenberg LE. A gender gap in the next generation of physician-scientists: medical student interest and participation in research. J Investig Med. 2002;50(6):7.
5. 6 Women Scientists Who Were Snubbed Due to Sexism. Culture. Published May 19, 2013. Accessed August 13, 2021. https://www.nationalgeographic.com/culture/article/130519-women-scientists-overlooked-dna-history-science.
6. Committee on Pediatric Research. Promoting education, mentorship, and support for pediatric research. Pediatrics. 2001;107(6):1447–50. https://doi.org/10.1542/peds.107.6.1447.
7. McCabe LL. National Institutes of Health support for research and training: future of pediatrician scientists. Arch Pediatr Adolesc Med. 1998;152(9):839–42. https://doi.org/10.1001/archpedi.152.9.839.
8. NIH Pediatric Research Consortium (N-PeRC). https://www.nichd.nih.gov/. Accessed August 13, 2021. https://www.nichd.nih.gov/research/supported/nperc.
9. Rivkees SA. The missing link of NIH funding in pediatric research training program restructuring. Pediatrics. 2014;134(6):e1521–2. https://doi.org/10.1542/peds.2014-1100.
10. Bowen CJ, Kersbergen CJ, Tang O, Cox A, Beach MC. Medical school research ranking is associated with gender inequality in MSTP application rates. BMC Med Educ. 2018;18(1):187. https://doi.org/10.1186/s12909-018-1306-z.
11. Gordon MB, Osganian SK, Emans SJ, Lovejoy FH. Gender differences in research Grant applications for pediatric residents. Pediatrics. 2009;124(2):e355–61. https://doi.org/10.1542/peds.2008-3626.
12. Gayet-Ageron A, Poncet A, Perneger T. Comparison of the contributions of female and male authors to medical research in 2000 and 2015: a cross-sectional study. BMJ Open. 2019;9(2):e024436. https://doi.org/10.1136/bmjopen-2018-024436.
13. Spector ND, Asante PA, Marcelin JR, et al. Women in pediatrics: progress, barriers, and opportunities for equity, diversity, and inclusion. Pediatrics. 2019;144(5):e20192149. https://doi.org/10.1542/peds.2019-2149.
14. Fishman M, Williams WA, Goodman DM, Ross LF. Gender differences in the authorship of original research in pediatric journals, 2001–2016. J Pediatr. 2017;191:244–249.e1. https://doi.org/10.1016/j.jpeds.2017.08.044.
15. Silver JK, Poorman JA, Reilly JM, Spector ND, Goldstein R, Zafonte RD. Assessment of women physicians among authors of perspective-type articles published in high-impact pediatric journals. JAMA Netw Open. 2018;1(3):e180802. https://doi.org/10.1001/jamanetworkopen.2018.0802.
16. Denby KJ, Szpakowski N, Silver J, Walsh MN, Nissen S, Cho L. Representation of women in cardiovascular clinical trial leadership. JAMA Intern Med. 2020;180(10):1382. https://doi.org/10.1001/jamainternmed.2020.2485.
17. Andersen JP, Nielsen MW, Simone NL, Lewiss RE, Jagsi R. COVID-19 medical papers have fewer women first authors than expected. eLife. 2020;9:e58807. https://doi.org/10.7554/eLife.58807.
18. Scholarly Activity | The American Board of Pediatrics. Accessed August 13, 2021. https://www.abp.org/content/scholarly-activity.
19. Voelker R. Robert wood Johnson clinical scholars mark 35 years of health services research. Medical News & Perspectives. 2007:2571–3.
20. National Clinician Scholars Program | NCSP National Clinician Scholars Program. Accessed August 13, 2021. https://nationalcsp.org/.

21. Steiner JF, Curtis P, Lanphear BP, Vu KO, Main DS. Assessing the role of influential mentors in the research development of primary care fellows. Acad Med J Assoc Am Med Coll. 2004;79(9):865–72. https://doi.org/10.1097/00001888-200409000-00012.
22. Saha S, Christakis DA, Saint S, Whooley MA, Simon SR. Perspectives a survival guide for generalist physicians in part 1. Getting Started. 1999;April
23. Sambuco D, Dabrowska A, DeCastro R, Stewart A, Ubel PA, Jagsi R. Negotiation in academic medicine: narratives of faculty researchers and their mentors. Acad Med. 2013;88(4):505–11. https://doi.org/10.1097/ACM.0b013e318286072b.
24. Saha S, Saint S, Christakis DA, Simon SR, Fihn SD. A survival guide for generalist physicians: preparing for the transition to junior faculty. J Gen Intern Med. 1999;April:750–5.
25. Connelly MT, Sullivan AM, Chinchilla M, et al. The impact of a junior faculty fellowship award on academic advancement and retention. Acad Med. 2017;92(8):1160–7. https://doi.org/10.1097/ACM.0000000000001541.
26. Sege R, Nykiel-Bub L, Selk S. Sex differences in institutional support for junior biomedical researchers. JAMA. 2015;314(11):1175. https://doi.org/10.1001/jama.2015.8517.
27. Carr PL. Relation of family responsibilities and gender to the productivity and career satisfaction of medical faculty. Ann Intern Med. 1998;129(7):532. https://doi.org/10.7326/0003-4819-129-7-199810010-00004.
28. Moreno MA, Katzenellenbogen R. Women rock science: a pocket guide for success in clinical academic research careers. Cham, Switzerland: Springer; 2019.
29. Alexander D, Boat T, Britto M, et al. Federation of Pediatric Organizations Task Force on women in pediatrics: considerations for part-time training and employment for research-intensive fellows and faculty. J Pediatr. 2009;154(1):1–3.e2. https://doi.org/10.1016/j.jpeds.2008.08.010.
30. Women Chairs of the Association of Medical School Pediatric Department Chairs. Women in pediatrics: recommendations for the future. Pediatrics. 2007;119(5):1000–5. https://doi.org/10.1542/peds.2006-2909.
31. Carr PL, Gunn CM, Kaplan SA, Raj A, Freund KM. Inadequate progress for women in academic medicine: findings from the National Faculty Study. J Women's Health. 2015;24(3):190–9. https://doi.org/10.1089/jwh.2014.4848.

Chapter 12
Networking, Mentorship, Sponsorship, Coaching, and Career Development Activities to Support Women in Pediatrics

Jennifer K. O'Toole, Barbara Overholser, and Nancy D. Spector

The Importance of Networking

Networking is the process of creating one's fabric of personal contacts who will provide support, feedback, insight, resources, information, and opportunities throughout one's career [21]. Many find networking insincere or manipulative, and women often suffer the consequences of having poorly developed professional networks. Building one's operational, personal, and strategic networks, which allow for adequate mentorship, sponsorship, coaching, and allyship, is vital to supporting a woman's career. It's been written that "the alternative to networking is to fail – either in reaching for a leadership position or in succeeding at it,"[21] and it is true. Those who invest time and effort in networking tend to be more successful in their careers than "those who fail to leverage external ties"[21]. Finding a good role model who is able to apply judgment and intuition in order to effectively and ethically network is a good way to build one's skills as a networker.

Ibarra and Hunter describe three distinct forms of networking, including operational, personal, and strategic, as key components of the evolution of leaders on

J. K. O'Toole (✉)
Internal Medicine-Pediatrics Residency Program, Departments of Internal Medicine and Pediatrics, University of Cincinnati College of Medicine, Cincinnati Children's Hospital Medical Center, Cincinnati, OH, USA
e-mail: jennifer.otoole@cchmc.org

B. Overholser
Drexel University College of Medicine, Executive Leadership in Academic Medicine® (ELAM), Philadelphia, PA, USA
e-mail: Bro29@drexel.edu

N. D. Spector
Executive Leadership in Academic Medicine® (ELAM), Office of Faculty, Drexel University College of Medicine, Philadelphia, PA, USA
e-mail: Nds24@drexel.edu

N. D. Spector et al. (eds.), *Women in Pediatrics*,
https://doi.org/10.1007/978-3-030-98222-5_12

Table 12.1 Types of networking

Type of networking	Operational networking	Personal networking	Strategic networking
Description	➤The development of relationships with the people who help you do your job, including direct reports, peers, supervisors, and key collaborators (usually internal). ➤Allows to get work done efficiently and is oriented around a task or goal. ➤Depth of the network and strong working relationships are key. ➤Focus – Internal	➤The development of relationships with individuals in professional organizations, affinity groups, and communities of interest external to one's primary team or organization. ➤Allows an individual to gain new perspectives, referrals, information, and developmental support. ➤Breadth of network and developing contacts who can make referrals is key. ➤Focus – External	➤The development of lateral and vertical relationships with other managers and leaders outside of one's control and institution. Provides the relationships and information to achieve personal and organizational goals. ➤Allows an individual to figure out future priorities and challenges and engage stakeholders. ➤Creating leverage with internal and external relationships is key. ➤Focus – Strategic, internal, and external

their quest to career advancement. These various forms of networking are described in Table 12.1. In their study of leaders who are seeking to build networking relationships, the authors found that operational networking helps to manage current responsibilities, personal networking helps to boost personal development, and strategic networking highlights future opportunities and directions [21].

It is important to note that women and men network differently, at different times and sometimes in different settings. Due to the paucity of women in leadership or the highest ranks in medicine and more specifically in pediatrics, women may need to look outside of their specialty, institution, or even discipline to find the needed support network and counsel they seek. Once women achieve leadership positions or success, they must then reach back and help those who are rising up the ranks. In order to change the landscape for future generations of women in medicine, it is imperative to create a network of women at the top who are willing to change the landscape and give other women the opportunities they were not afforded.

Mentorship

In academic medicine, effective mentorship is considered one of the most important determinants of success [36]. Yet women underinvest in key social capital opportunities to establish and maintain mentorship relationships, leaving them at a disadvantage [16]. For women with intersectional identities, mentorship and sponsorship are even more crucial to ensure access to opportunities, achievement of success, and advancement. Tsedale M. Melaku's research has shown that sponsorship is "critical to Black women's access to significant training, development, and networking opportunities and advancement" [25]. While Chap. 10 speaks to the importance of male allyship in supporting women in pediatrics, it's important to note that to really optimize a culture of support for all women, we need to additionally consider how white women should serve as mentors and critical allies for women with intersectionality. "Only 10 percent of Black women and 19 percent of Latinas say the majority of their strongest allies are white, compared to 45 percent of white women" [34]. In order to achieve true equity for all women in pediatrics, white women need to step forward and serve as mentors and key allies for women of color.

A mentor is an experienced and trusted advisor, typically in one's own field, who uses their knowledge and experience to counsel [23]. Typically, mentorship occurs in a dyadic fashion between a more senior and junior individual, in which the senior mentor provides wisdom, guidance, and support. However, there are various other types of mentoring relationships that are critical to the success of women in medicine. Table 12.2 highlights various types of mentoring relationships that women in medicine often participate in.

Table 12.2 Types of mentoring relationships

Type of mentoring	Description
Traditional dyadic mentoring [27]	➤Most common type of mentoring. Pairs one mentor with one mentee in which the mentor is more senior in experience ➤Mentor and mentee develop a relationship in which the mentor provides guidance and support ➤Accountability may be based upon formal contracts between mentor and mentee
Functional mentoring [31]	➤Pairs a mentee with a mentor with specific expertise for guidance on a distinct project ➤Objectives are clearly defined and lead to tangible results ➤There are timelines and deadlines that the mentee must adhere to
Peer mentoring	➤Individuals at similar level, stage, or position provide mentoring ➤Provide advice and support given similar lived experience, however may lack time and experience ➤No defined results or outcomes
Situational mentoring	➤Mentoring for a specific purpose/skill or to assist in achieving a particular outcome ➤Common at all stages of the career
Facilitate group mentoring [22]	➤Centers the group members as peer mentors to each other ➤Senior person facilitates the process ➤Mentees work collaboratively and have formal goals and objectives
Supervisory mentoring [27]	➤Advisor as mentor and direct supervisor ➤Not all supervisors are comfortable also being a mentor ➤Possibility of conflict of interest
Speed mentoring [28]	➤Setup is similar to "speed dating" in which one mentee gets to meet with various mentors in a back-to-back format for short periods of time ➤Facilitated by a central source ➤While initial sessions are short, mentees and mentors gain introductions that allow for future connections

Diversity in one's mentorship team is important for women in pediatrics. Mentors of different genders, races, and ethnicities and from inside and outside one's organization can offer broader perspectives to challenges. In pediatrics and in most other areas of medicine, men hold the most powerful leadership positions. In order to achieve gender equity, it's imperative that these men support women's advancement by being mentors. Women in pediatrics need to prioritize mentoring by actively engaging in networking as outlined above to actively seek and secure mentors.

> "*People have amazing promise and potential. Each has a unique light within. Mentoring is a privilege, a special trust bringing us closer to another's nascent spark and the heat at their core. Mentoring is also a generational charge, a responsibility to protect that light, to shield it, nurture it, help another learn how to tend to and control the fire so that it may fuel dreams, collaborations, and change.*" – Judy Schaechter, MD, MBA, President and Chief Executive Officer of the American Board of Pediatrics.

Pediatric physician-scientists have their own unique needs for mentorship, as Dr. Sallie Permar, chair of the Department of Pediatrics at Weill Cornell Medicine and pediatrician-in-chief at NewYork-Presbyterian/Weill Cornell Medical Center and NewYork-Presbyterian Komansky Children's Hospital describes:

> "*Mentorship is critical in all aspects of academic medicine, but particularly in areas that lack representation in academic medicine leadership from the populations we serve. In particular, pediatricians are underrepresented in academic medicine leadership, and it is the interest of children and their future health that may suffer in that setting. Thus, structured mentorship of diverse future pediatrician and pediatrician-scientist leaders is critical to the trajectory of the health of our nation and globe.*
>
> *Pediatrician-scientists are a specific group that are underrepresented among physician-scientists and declining in number, jeopardizing advancement in cures and prevention of childhood diseases, as well as addressing the origins of costly adult diseases. A disparity in the representation of children's health in the portfolio of funded physician investigators is a threat to our achievements in lifelong health. Yet the pipeline of pediatric physician scientists is threatened by ballooning medical education debt and relatively low salaries in the field of pediatrics that typically support research, a concentration of pediatric research funding at a small number of large institutions, and a declining number and aging population of mentors.*
>
> *Pipeline efforts are vital to ensuring progress in basic and translational discoveries that yield improved lifelong health are reliant on mentorship, a key tenant of academic medicine. Mentoring of future pediatrician-leaders and scientists who represent all backgrounds is how we promise a healthier future to our children and the adults they will become.*"

Sponsorship

While mentoring is a central component of the leadership journey, sponsorship is more focused on advancement, power, and accelerating the career trajectory, and in many ways, it is more vital for women than mentorship. Some research has shown that having a mentor increases the likelihood of promotion for men, but not for women, perhaps because women's mentors tend to be less senior that those of their colleagues who are men and therefore don't have adequate influence to advocate for them [20].

Sponsorship is defined as the "public support by a powerful, influential person for the advancement and promotion of an individual within whom he or she sees untapped or unappreciated leadership talent or potential"[20]. It is also characterized by its bi-directionality: the sponsor and protégé share values and offer each other complementary skill sets. Sponsors have the clout to advocate for a promotion in a public way, connect protégés with senior leaders, come to their aid when their protégé is in trouble, and call in favors on their behalf [19]. A protégé supports their sponsor's passion and promotes their legacy. They then pay it forward by becoming sponsors themselves.

For women, sponsorship is critically important. For women of color, in particular, sponsorship is an essential component to allow access to significant training, development, and networking opportunities and advancement [20]. But fewer women than men have sponsors. Why is that the case? Unconscious bias on the part of sponsors may play a role as well as women's underinvestment in seeking sponsors. And it may also be "the similarity principle" as Herminia Ibarra categorizes it:

> "*Here human nature creates an uneven playing field: People's tendency to gravitate to those who are like them on salient dimensions such as gender increases the likelihood that powerful men will sponsor and advocate for other men when leadership opportunities arise*" [20].

Institutions have an opportunity to close the sponsorship gap by building a strong internal culture of sponsorship by supporting and developing internal sponsorship programs. With a guiding set of principles to ground it, including training regarding gender and race issues, the sponsorship program can have tremendous impact. Magrane et al. have developed an instrument for self- and organizational assessment of mentoring and sponsorship practices leaders in academic engineering use [24]. This assessment has been adapted for academic health science faculty (Fig. 12.1) and can be useful for institutions seeking to develop intentional approaches to leadership development.

Career/Professional Development Programs

Career/professional development refers to training an individual may participate in with the goal to evolve, improve, or develop their professional skills, often associated with advancement within their given career path. Local and national career development programs have been found to have a positive impact on the promotion and advancement of women in medicine. Women who participate in these types of programs were noted to have greater career satisfaction, improved professional skills (e.g., interpersonal, leadership, negotiation, and networking skills), greater success in being promoted, a more rapid pace to promotion, and lower attrition rates in academic medicine [7, 8, 12, 18, 26].

We encourage women to actively think about pursuing career/professional development at all stages of their career. In selecting a program, women must be strategic and consider timing and skills needed and identify opportunities or challenges they

Leadership Mentoring & Sponsoring Self-Assessment for Academic Health Science Faculty

Reflect on how often you engage in the following practices and how you might facilitate additional sponsorship.
* Note that some mentoring practices can be sponsorship if they are and funded.

As a MENTOR, to what extent do you:	Rarely	Sometimes	Often	How could you do more?
1. Provide your mentee/protege with candid feedback.				
2. Discuss strategies for managing Interpersonal politics.				
3. Encourage attendance at internal or external leadership programs. *				
4. Seek feedback as to how he/she Is doing in the new leadership position.				
5. Set aside meetings on your calendar for regular mentoring.				
6. Advise her/him on executive presence and communications. 7. Guide her/him in development of an Intentional and strategic plan for advancement to leadership.				
8. *Provide opportunity to shadow you.				
As a MENTOR, to what extent do you:	**Rarely**	**Sometimes**	**Often**	**How could you do more?**
1. Publicly acknowledge her/his talents and achievements.				
2. Publicly support when he/she makes a difficult or unpopular decision.				
3. Appoint to internal or external high-level committees/task forces.				
4. Directly nominate her/him for advancement and prestigious positions.				
5. Assign her/him to an administrative role that tests new management skills, especially those with profit and loss responsibility. 6. Introduce her/him to individuals or groups to extend his/her professional networks.				
7. Send in your place to important meetings, speaking appearances, and events.				
8. Provide opportunities to present to executive groups (e.g., board meetings).				
9. Pave the entry to leadership by preparing other faculty for the new leader's role.				
10. Provide funding and resources for leadership program participation and/or leadership coaching.				
11. Engage a team of advisors and consultants to support the protege.				
12. Advocate with colleagues to advance protege				

Adapted from Magrane D, Morahan PS, Ambrose S, Dannels S, Competencies and Practices in Academic Engineering Leadership Development: Lessons from a National Survey. Soc. 2018, 7,171; doi:10.3390/socsci7100171

Fig. 12.1 Leadership mentoring and sponsoring self-assessment for academic health science faculty [24]

are currently facing or anticipate in their career. As one begins looking at development opportunities, individuals must also reflect on how they will apply the knowledge and skills from the program they are considering to their current position.

Women should also actively pursue support for these programs from their institution or employer. Supporting employees or faculty members in obtaining additional career/professional development is an excellent return on investment for institutions for their workforce becomes more skilled, productive, and has a higher likelihood retention.

Table 12.3 details some sample career development programs for women in medicine. Please note this is not an exhaustive list and programs may evolve with time. Rather, this is a list of programs that were well established at the time of publication of this book and are illustrative of the programs that many women in pediatrics have elected to attend.

We would like to highlight two career development programs for women in medicine that have proven impact. The ELAM® program at Drexel University College of Medicine is a prime example of a well-established and extremely successful national professional development program for mid- to senior-level women in academic medicine [17]. The program is a longitudinal part-time fellowship that focuses on expanding the national pool of qualified women candidates for leadership in academic medicine, dentistry, public health, and pharmacy and aims to ensure that there is gender equity at every level of leadership. The curriculum of this program is designed to address four fundamental competencies, including (1) strategic finance and resource management, (2) personal and professional leadership effectiveness, (3) organizational dynamics, and (4) communities of leadership practice. Since 1995, more than 1200 women have graduated from the program and have gone on to lead in high-level positions including as provosts, presidents, deans, and chairs at institutions and organizations around the country and the world. Roughly 140 of the alumnae are in the field of pediatrics, 27 of whom are chairs of their department.

The ELAM program is extremely successful because it makes use of its strong national alumnae network, incorporating them as faculty, mentors, and coaches for the current fellows. The program employs functional and facilitated peer group mentoring as part of the program's experiential learning process and also within small learning communities of six program fellows facilitated by one senior individual who is usually a graduate of the program. The benefits go in

Table 12.3 Example career/professional development programs

Local programs	Duke LEADER (Leadership Development for Researchers) Program [14] Wake Forest School of Medicine Early Career Development Program for Women [12] Drexel University Faculty Launch Program [13]
Specialty-based national programs	APPD LEAD [6] Advancing Pediatric Leaders [4] Society of Hospital Medicine Leadership Academy [29]
Cross-disciplinary national programs	Executive Leadership In Academic Medicine® (ELAM®) Program [17] AAMC Leadership Development Programs [2, 3]

Note this is not an exhaustive list, rather some illustrative programs

several ways – the fellows receive guidance and support from their peers and their advisor. The advisor receives enrichment from the fellows and returns to her home institution with new outlooks and perspectives. Programs such as ELAM are critically important for women in medicine, and leaders and mentors in pediatrics should strongly encourage and sponsor women at their institution to attend the program.

The Wake Forest School of Medicine (WFSM) Career Development for Women Leaders (CDWL) is a local, competitive program developed for mid- and senior-level women faculty who are in leadership roles or aspire to be leaders, as well as women staff at the VP level of healthcare administration [33]. This program was created in 2008 as the result of an ELAM's fellow Institutional Action Project, and 13 classes have completed the program for a total of 245 program graduates as of June 2021. Offered over 9 months, women attend one full-day session per month. It is an affordable, local option that allows more women to participate in leadership education. Women from diverse professional backgrounds from multiple institutions including WFSM, Wake Forest University, and surrounding universities come to the program to exchange ideas and foster cross-campus collaboration.

The program modules mirror many of ELAM's and include team building, institutional finances, decision-making strategies for leaders, and creating and sustaining diversity. CDWL's internal data reports that 56% of the 245 program graduates have accepted a new leadership role, and of those, 36% accepted more than one new leadership role. Nineteen percent of 245 CDWL program graduates have left their institution, and of those, 52% left for bigger leadership roles at new institutions [10].

Professional Coaching

Another critical resource in helping women to advance, overcome barriers, and achieve their full potential in medicine is professional coaching. Coaches provide specific instruction, assist at increasing performance at work, and assist with professional development. They are not sounding boards; they help clarify goals, ask for intentional actions and behaviors, and keep their clients accountable and on track with their plans. For those earlier in their career, executive coaching has been found to effectively reduce physician burnout, which impacts women more than men [5] – women have a 60 percent greater odds of reporting burnout compared with men – and is a phenomenon that has only increased during the COVID-19 pandemic and its continuing aftermath. Dyrbye et al. conducted a pilot trial for professional coaching for 88 physicians at Mayo Clinic sites and found that coaching can be an effective intervention for addressing burnout and quality of life and can aid in building resilience and that developing a formal, institutionally sponsored professional coaching experience can improve physician well-being [15]. For people further along in their career, professional coaches can help with transitions into leadership positions.

Controlling Your Own Destiny

As women in pediatrics seek to build their networks, create their mentorship team, and find strategic sponsors, they must also recognize that *they* are the most important person in determining the path to success. During medical school, residency, and fellowship training, built-in support and mentorship structures help to provide critical guideposts in one's career development. However, once training ends, women often find themselves floundering in a vast new world. While many practices and institutions have some infrastructure for career or faculty development and mentorship, it is never to the level that one finds in training. Therefore, it is critical that women recognize the importance of having a strong sense of responsibility for their success while they capitalize upon the structures that exist for their own development and advancement.

While we must create pediatric healthcare institutions that support women in their development and advancement, women must be the main driver of their success. Women must ensure they are driving their mentoring experience by managing up, setting an agenda, and asking for the things they need [11]. Mentors and sponsors who are more senior in their career are often very busy and have limited time. Therefore, women in pediatrics must maximize their time and asks from their mentors and sponsors by setting agendas for meetings, making realistic asks of them, and learning how they can most effectively and efficiently get what they need from them [9]. Women must deliver on their assigned or promised tasks, and project eagerness and excitement to be a part of the mentoring relationship. Regardless of their temperament, preferred communication style, and comfort with building networks, they must invest in the social capital of developing and maintaining strong local and national networks. Women in pediatrics must ask mentors and sponsors to create connections to key people in their area of interest or who can create opportunities for them in the future.

As women rise in leadership or higher academic ranks, it is their responsibility to intentionally reach out to women joining the field and provide assistance, advice, and sponsorship. Even if these senior women were not afforded appropriate mentorship, sponsorship, or networking opportunities early in their career, they must change the narrative and create a culture where we "lift others as we rise." Women in senior positions in pediatrics must continually ask themselves who needs to be lifted up, whose voice needs to be heard or amplified, and who needs to be given a chance at a new opportunity. In order to truly change the destiny for women in pediatrics, women must support one another, create networks, sponsor each other, and find power in collaboration. As Shelley Zalis stated, "*There is a special place in heaven for women who support other women*" [35].

References

1. AAMC. 2018–2019 The State of Women in Academic Medicine: Exploring Pathways to Equity. 2018–2019. Retrieved September 20, 2021 from https://www.aamc.org/data-reports/data/2018-2019-state-women-academic-medicine-exploring-pathways-equity.
2. AAMC Early Career Women Faculty Leadership Development Seminar. Retrieved October 20, 2021 from https://www.aamc.org/professional-development/leadership-development/ewims.
3. AAMC Mid-Career Women Faculty Leadership Development Seminar. Retrieved October 21, 2021 from https://www.aamc.org/professional-development/leadership-development/midwims.
4. Advancing Pediatric Leaders. Retrieved October 20, 2021 from https://www.academicpeds.org/programs-awards/advancing-pediatric-leaders/.
5. Alexander L, Bonnema R, Farmer S, Reimold S. Executive coaching women faculty: a focused strategy to build resilience. Phys Leadership J. 2020;7(1):41–4.
6. APPD Leadership in Educational Academic Development (LEAD). Retrieved October 20, 2021 from https://www.appd.org/resources-programs/educational-resources/appd-lead/.
7. Chang S, Guindani M, Morahan P, Magrane D, Newbill S, Helitzer D. Increasing promotion of women Faculty in Academic Medicine: impact of National Career Development Programs. J Womens Health (Larchmt). 2020;29(6):837–46. https://doi.org/10.1089/jwh.2019.8044.
8. Chang S, Morahan PS, Magrane D, Helitzer D, Lee HY, Newbill S, Cardinali G. Retaining Faculty in Academic Medicine: the impact of career development programs for women. J Womens Health (Larchmt). 2016;25(7):687–96. https://doi.org/10.1089/jwh.2015.5608.
9. Chopra V, Saint S. What mentors wish their mentees knew. 2017. https://hbr.org/2017/11/what-mentors-wish-their-mentees-knew.
10. Correspondence from Wake Forest School of Medicine WIMS Career and Leadership Development Programs. November 2021.
11. Cruz M, Bhatia D, Calaman S, Dickinson B, Dreyer B, Frost M, Spector N.. The Mentee-Driven Approach to Mentoring Relationships and Career Success: Benefits for Mentors and Mentees. *MedEdPORTAL*. 2015, 11. https://doi.org/10.15766/mep_2374-8265.10201.
12. Danhauer SC, Tooze JA, Barrett NA, Blalock JS, Shively CA, Voytko ML, Crandall SJ. Development of an innovative career development program for early-career women faculty. Glob Adv Health Med. 2019;8:2164956119862986. https://doi.org/10.1177/2164956119862986.
13. Drexel University College of Medicine Faculty Launch Program. Retrieved October 15, 2021 from https://drexel.edu/medicine/faculty-and-staff/faculty-and-staff-resources/faculty-launch-program/.
14. Duke University School of Medicine LEADER Program. Retrieved October 15, 2021 from https://medschool.duke.edu/about-us/faculty-resources/faculty-development/our-programs/leadership-development-researchers.
15. Dyrbye LN, Shanafelt TD, Gill PR, Satele DV, West CP. Effect of a professional coaching intervention on the well-being and distress of physicians: a pilot randomized clinical trial. JAMA Intern Med. 2019;179(10):1406–14. https://doi.org/10.1001/jamainternmed.2019.2425.
16. Eagly A, Carli L. Women and the Labyrinth of Leadership. 2007. Retrieved November 1, 2021 from https://hbr.org/2007/09/women-and-the-labyrinth-of-leadership.
17. Executive Leadership in Academic Medicine program. Retrieved October 7, 2021 from https://drexel.edu/medicine/academics/womens-health-and-leadership/elam/.
18. Helitzer DL, Newbill SL, Morahan PS, Magrane D, Cardinali G, Wu CC, Chang S. Perceptions of skill development of participants in three national career development programs for women faculty in academic medicine. Acad Med. 2014;89(6):896–903. https://doi.org/10.1097/ACM.0000000000000251.
19. Hewlett SA. The sponsor effect: how to be a better leader by investing in others. Harvard Business Review Press; 2019.

20. Ibarra H. A lack of Sponsorship is Keeping Women from Advancing into Leadership. 2019. Retrieved October 7, 2021 from https://hbr.org/2019/08/a-lack-of-sponsorship-is-keeping-women-from-advancing-into-leadership.
21. Ibarra H, Hunter ML. How Leaders Create and Use Networks. Harvard Business Review. 2007. Retrieved September 20, 2021 from https://hbr.org/2007/01/how-leaders-create-and-use-networks.
22. Kuzma N, Skuby S, Souder E, Cruz M, Dickinson B, Spector N, Calaman S. Reflect, advise, plan: faculty-facilitated peer-group mentoring to optimize individualized learning plans. Acad Pediatr. 2016;16(6):503–7. https://doi.org/10.1016/j.acap.2016.06.002.
23. Loethen J, Ananthamurugan M. Women in medicine: the quest for mentorship. Mo Med. 2021;118(3):182–4.
24. Magrane D, Morahan PS, Ambrose S, Dannels SA. Competencies and practices in academic engineering leadership development: lessons from a National Survey. Soc Sci. 2018;7(10):171.
25. Melaku T, Beeman A, Smith D, Johnson WB. Be a Better ALly. Harvard Business Review. 2020. Retrieved September 20, 2021 from https://hbr.org/2020/11/be-a-better-ally.
26. Nowling TK, McClure E, Simpson A, Sheidow AJ, Shaw D, Feghali-Bostwick C. A focused career development program for women faculty at an academic medical center. J Womens Health (Larchmt). 2018;27(12):1474–81. https://doi.org/10.1089/jwh.2018.6937.
27. Raluca C. How many types of mentoring are there? 2020. Retrieved October 7, 2021 from https://blog.matrixlms.com/how-many-types-of-mentoring-are-there/.
28. Serwint JR, Cellini MM, Spector ND, Gusic ME. The value of speed mentoring in a pediatric academic organization. Acad Pediatr. 2014;14(4):335–40. https://doi.org/10.1016/j.acap.2014.02.009.
29. Society of Hospital Medicine's Leadership Academy. Retrieved October 20, 2021 from https://www.hospitalmedicine.org/event/leadership-academy/.
30. Spector ND, Overholser B. Leadership and professional development: sponsored; catapulting underrepresented talent off the cusp and into the game. J Hosp Med. 2019;14(7):415. https://doi.org/10.12788/jhm.3214
31. Thorndyke LE, Gusic ME, Milner RJ. Functional mentoring: a practical approach with multilevel outcomes. J Contin Educ Heal Prof. 2008;28(3):157–64. https://doi.org/10.1002/chp.178.
32. Travis EL, Doty L, Helitzer DL. Sponsorship: a path to the academic medicine C-suite for women faculty? Acad Med. 2013;88(10):1414–7. https://doi.org/10.1097/ACM.0b013e3182a35456.
33. Wake Forest School of Medicine Career Development for Women Leaders Program. Retrieved October 19, 2021 from https://school.wakehealth.edu/About-the-School/Faculty-Affairs/Faculty-Development/Women-in-Medicine-and-Science/Career-Development.
34. White employees see themselves as allies—but Black women and Latinas disagree. Retrieved December 20, 2021 from https://leanin.org/research/allyship-at-work.
35. Zalis S. Power of the Pack: Women Who Support Women are more Successful. 2019. https://www.forbes.com/sites/shelleyzalis/2019/03/06/power-of-the-pack-women-who-support-women-are-more-successful/?sh=cb454ac1771a.
36. Zerzan JT, Hess R, Schur E, Phillips RS, Rigotti N. Making the most of mentors: a guide for mentees. Acad Med. 2009;84(1):140–4. https://doi.org/10.1097/ACM.0b013e3181906e8f.

Chapter 13
Advocacy Efforts in Pediatrics

Advocating for the Most Vulnerable Part of Population that Has No Voice

Anika Kumar and Pam Shaw

> Advocacy is in the DNA of Pediatricians. – Mark DelMonte JD, CEO of the American Academy of Pediatrics (2018–present)

History of Advocacy in Pediatrics

The American Medical Association's (AMA's) Section on Diseases of Children was formally established in 1880 by pediatricians, including Abraham Jacobi, MD, a legacy leader in the field of pediatrics. He advocated for access to birth control, the admission of women to Johns Hopkins School of Medicine, and the advancement of minority communities. The American Pediatric Society (APS) was established in 1888. Although the AMA's Section on Diseases of Children and the APS were involved in research and scholarly work, they were not involved in advocacy in an organized fashion. Neither organization believed that pediatricians should be involved in social or political activities [3].

Early pediatricians were advocates for pasteurization of milk and prevention of infectious disease. In the early 1900s, pediatricians became advocates for

---

Advocating for the Most Vulnerable Part of Population that Has No Voice

---

A. Kumar (✉)
Cleveland Clinic Lerner College of Medicine of Case Western Reserve University, Cleveland, OH, USA
e-mail: KumarA4@ccf.org

P. Shaw
University of Kansas School of Medicine, Kansas City, KS, USA
e-mail: PSHAW@kumc.edu

N. D. Spector et al. (eds.), *Women in Pediatrics*,
https://doi.org/10.1007/978-3-030-98222-5_13

improving the status of children. Early pediatricians believed then, as we do today, that childhood is the period of life that impacts adulthood and by addressing poverty and childhood trauma, children would become healthier adults. The child welfare leaders were in organizations known as the US Children's Bureau and the Bureau of Child Hygiene. The Bureau of Child Hygiene was led by a pediatrician named Dr. S. Josephine Baker. By working at a health department from 1908 to 1914, Dr. Baker reduced infant mortality in New York City by using visiting nurses and promoting breastfeeding to improve conditions for infants. All this work reached a climax in 1921 with the passage of the Sheppard-Towner Maternity and Infancy Protection Act. The Sheppard-Towner Act provided just over $1 million dollars in matching funds for states to set up programs promoting infant health and visiting nurses. The AMA condemned the act as "state medicine" and intrusion of government into private practice. Sheppard-Towner expired in 1929 because of active opposition from organized medicine, including the AMA. This opposition of investment in the lives of women and children by the AMA led to an important meeting in 1929 to establish another organization [3].

In 1929, during a meeting of the AMA's Section on Diseases of Children, 35 pediatricians gathered at a private home of one of the members. The members there began the discussion of creating a new organization for all practicing pediatricians. They suggested the name the American Academy of Pediatrics (AAP). The organization was officially founded in July of 1930 in Illinois. There were three women charter members of the organization. By the 1940s, women made up 13% of pediatricians and 3.5% of general practitioners [3].

Meanwhile, Dr. Martha Eliot and Dr. Katherine Bain were both pioneers in advocacy at the Children's Bureau. In 1934, Dr. Eliot participated in drafting Title V of the Social Security Act, which revived the maternal and child measures of the Sheppard-Towner Act, and continues to support maternal and child health today. Dr. Eliot, a pioneer in advocacy, took over at the US Children's Bureau in 1939. She helped envision a national study of health services for children in 1945. In 1949, the Commonwealth Fund published the data that provided a comprehensive picture of pediatric practitioners, children's hospitals, and the curricula about pediatrics in 70 medical schools [3].

At the 1953 meeting of the American Pediatric Society and Society for Pediatric Research (APS-SPR), Dr. Barbara Korsch convened an informal group to discuss the importance of ambulatory care. This led to the formation of the Association for Ambulatory Pediatric Services in 1960. One of the tenets of the new organization was active participation of the membership. "Advocacy became fairly early an important issue…We didn't have a structure to really advocate at the national level very effectively, but we were taking positions all the time and issuing statements" [22]. The current Academic Pediatric Association (APA) was established in 2007 with a name change.

The AAP appointed a committee on legislation in 1935 to track legislation and work with the federal government, but the legislative advocacy began in earnest when the Washington, DC office was established in 1970. Major legislation in the 1970s included the Lead-Based Paint Poisoning Prevention Act, which required Health and Human Services to prohibit lead-based paint in residential structures. Dr. Herbert Needleman identified and published about the dangers of lead and specifically lead-based paint in the 1950s which led to the legislation mentioned above after years of fighting the lead companies [3].

In 1973, the APA elected its first woman president, Dr. Katherine S. Lobach. From 1970 to 1980, medical schools saw a 60% increase in enrollment and for the first-time women made inroads. The percent of women entering medical school went from 11% in 1970 to 29% by 1980.

The Omnibus Reconciliation Act (OBRA) of 1981 was passed with major cuts to domestic programs. Cuts in Aid to Families with Dependent Children (AFDC) and Medicaid caused a major increase in the number of uninsured children. This became a major advocacy opportunity for pediatricians to promote preventive care and a minimum benefits package for Medicaid. In 1982, a sensationalized TV report "DPT: Vaccine Roulette" was aired and threatened the vaccine supply in the United States. This soon became another advocacy opportunity for the pediatric community to rally around. In 1984, the AAP invited the APA, APS, SPR, and the Association of Medical School Pediatric Department Chairs to join the AAP's Committee on Federal Government Affairs to work on public policy issues together [3].

More women entered medical school and represented 39% of first year students by 1990. By 1990, 54% of pediatric residents were women. The proportion of all residents who were underrepresented remained unchanged over the decade, as only 11% were Black, Indigenous, and People of Color (BIPOC). In 1990, the AAP elected their first woman president, Dr. Antoinette Eaton. The 1990s were also a time when two women pediatricians served as US Surgeon Generals, Dr. Antonia Novello and Dr. M. Joycelyn Elders [3].

The 1990s were also marked by issues related to access to care and child health financing. The Vaccines for Children program paved the way to provide for vaccines in pediatricians' offices at no cost for low income and Medicaid children. Dr. Betty Lowe was the AAP president in 1993 and advocated in Washington to develop this popular program [3]. A major achievement, now known as the State Children's Health Insurance Program (SCHIP), was passed, allowing federal matching funds to be given to states to provide health coverage to children who did not qualify for Medicaid and did not have private insurance [3].

In 2009, the reauthorization of SCHIP occurred after being vetoed the previous year and was renamed the Children's Health Insurance Program (CHIP). The next milestone in insurance occurred in 2010 with the adoption of the Affordable Care Act (ACA). The AAP also elected its first Black president in 2007, Dr. Renee Jenkins [3].

From 2010 to present day, there have been many advocacy successes that are remarkable including the National Institutes of Health allowing children to be included in research via the Twenty-First Century Cures Act. Starting in 2016, the AAP began publishing the "Blueprint for Children" designed to guide the federal government on how best to improve children's health. The plan outlines specific child health goals and actionable policy recommendations for the US Federal Government and highlights the AAP's priorities for the upcoming 2–4 years. Since that time, the AAP has revised and updated the document during election years, including both presidential and mid-term elections. Many AAP state chapters have adopted similar "State Blueprints for Children" for gubernatorial transitions [19].

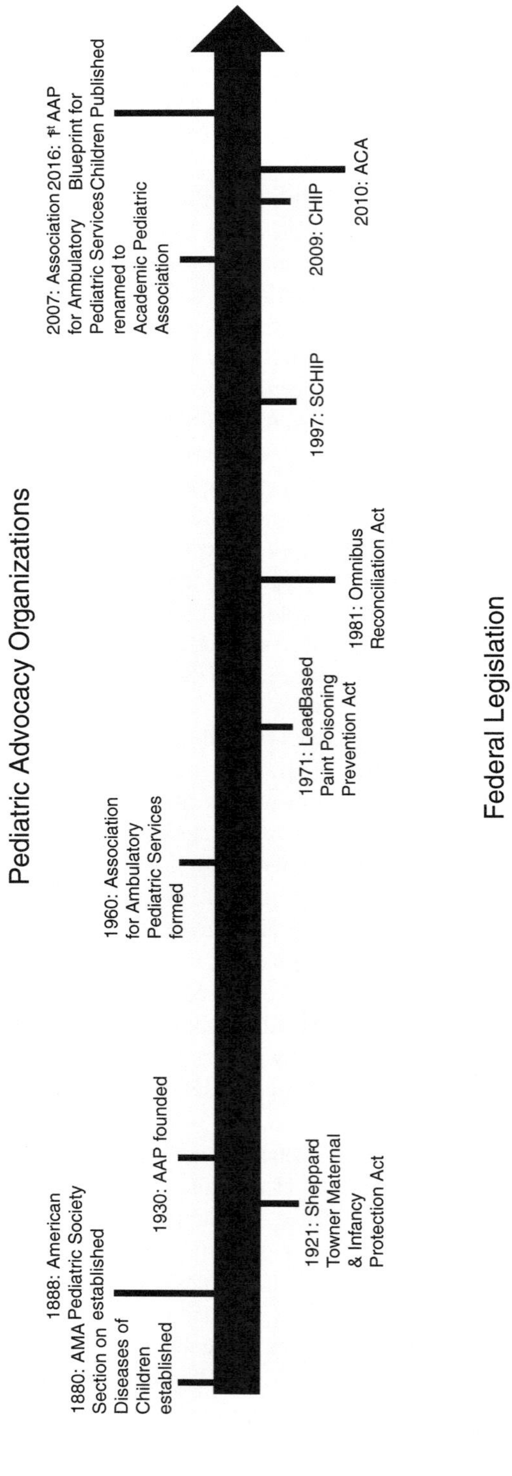

Fig. 13.1 Timeline of pediatric advocacy organizations and important child health federal legislation

Present day, women pediatricians are leaders in advocacy as committee chairs and presidents of pediatric organizations and in their offices. All the pediatric leadership organizations have come full circle and are involved in the social and political areas for the children in our country (Fig. 13.1).

Advocacy Training

One of the competencies for medical students, residents, and physicians is professionalism. Professionalism in pediatrics encourages advocacy on behalf of society and their patients.

Since 2001, the Accreditation Council for Graduate Medical Education (ACGME) Pediatric Residency Review Committee has required that pediatric residency programs provide educational experiences that prepare residents for the role of advocate for the health of children within the community. According to a systematic review of the literature [13], advocacy curricula is offered in many specialties, with 84% in primary care. Of these primary care residencies, pediatric residencies made up most of the primary care residencies that had formal curricula and objectives related to advocacy. The premise that requiring knowledge, skills, and attitudes about advocacy will enable a resident to advocate effectively is a strong one. The most common facilitators for advocacy curriculum include support from leadership; protected faculty time; direct funding, such as the Anne E. Dyson Community Pediatrics Training Initiative, or funding from the medical school; and the availability of resources and skills within the faculty and community. Dr. Anne E. Dyson, as a pediatrician, was committed to improving the lives of children. With her leadership of the Dyson Foundation, she was able to provide financial support to expand medical services and community involvement [20]. Other facilitators for advocacy include formal collaboration with a professional organization such as the state chapters of the AAP with a specialty-specific curriculum.

The most common barriers to organized advocacy are competing time demands and conflicts with clinical responsibilities. The lack of faculty champions and turnover also contribute to barriers for successful advocacy programs. The need for faculty champions and faculty who are skillful in advocacy are major drivers, and advocacy should be considered a skill that can help faculty be successful as teachers and clinicians, and help with promotion or success in their clinical efforts.

There are training opportunities for medical students, residents, faculty, and physicians in the community. The AAP hosts a yearly conference to teach advocacy skills and give participants an opportunity to practice these skills with Capitol Hill visits in Washington, DC. Skilled faculty present workshops and teach and role-play how to advocate for children and families.

As mentioned above, the state chapters of the AAP often partner with resideny training programs to have a legislative day or advocacy day during which residents, faculty, and community physicians are briefed on state child health issues and make legislative visits at their state capitals. This is a great way for resident physicians to understand the basic skills needed in speaking with their lawmakers.

The APA has also been involved in helping increase the skills of young faculty with the establishment of the Health Policy Scholars Program (HPSP) in 2020. This program is led by three dynamic women leaders: Dr. Lois Lee, Dr. Lenore Jarvis, and Dr. Lauren Gambill. This three-year faculty development program is designed to educate APA members on the development of a systematic and scholarly approach to health policy and advocacy. The primary goal of the APA's HPSP is to prepare scholars for a successful academic career in public policy and advocacy through mentorship, networking, and designing projects that meet the standards for professional review. The goal is to provide the academic background needed for promotion for those pediatricians who are in an academic program and need research and scholarly work.

Many examples of advocacy begin as educational programs or community service. One of these examples includes lead poisoning and its effect on childhood development. Historically, approaches to lead-based paint have been reactive in responding to a lead-poisoned child, rather than preventative. In 1971 there was national legislation which focused on reacting when a lead-poisoned child was identified and covered the cost of replacing the lead-based paint, which was most likely the cause. In 1992, Title X was created to reduce the sources of lead including lead-based paint before children were poisoned. This legislation also included other sources of lead, such as dust and soil. The research on lead and its hazard to children were responsible for the change in prevalence and the change in the focus to try to prevent lead damage to the developing brain. This led to a more contemporary focus on lead in Flint, Michigan [3].

A pediatrician in Flint, Dr. Mona Hanna-Attisha noticed that many of her patients had high lead levels. She used state and local databases to prove that the children of Flint had been exposed to lead in the water pipes when the local water supply was changed by the government. She used her advocacy and research skills to prove there was a problem, and brought the problem to the attention of public health officials and the local and state government to bring about change [12].

The most successful advocacy is often accomplished with partnerships between public health and epidemiology. The identification of a public health problem or issue can be the seed that leads to advocacy to change the underlying issues or obtain a grant to provide support or intervention to change the underlying problem.

Advocacy can also include working with local, state, or federal government, that often has to evolve to be successful. One example would be car seat safety and legislation. Originally "child seats" started out as nothing more than burlap sacks with a drawstring that hung over the headrest on the passenger's seat. Later, in 1933, manufacturers produced a seat that was basically a booster seat. It took until 1962 before people considered car seats as possible safety devices. It took an additional 9 years from the innovation of safety conscious car seats before regulations for safety were developed. In 1971, the National Highway Traffic Safety Administration adopted the first federal standards. At that time requirements did not include crash tests, but did require the use of a safety belt to hold the car seat onto the vehicle and a harness to hold the child in the car seat. It took an additional 17 years from innovation and 8 years from preliminary regulations until the first state law was enacted. It took another 6 years until all the states had laws. Leaders in child seat safety include Dr. Marilyn Bull, a developmental pediatrician, who spent her career advocating for car seat safety, especially for children with developmental concerns. Car seat safety is still evolving as research and innovation continue to make changes possible to keep children safe in cars [22].

Another area that effects young children that is evolving is firearm safety. As car safety has shown, it can be a long process to get to the finish line with legislation that makes gun safety a priority. Dr. Katherine Christoffel spent more than 20 years doing research, writing, and speaking out forcefully against violence, especially gun violence. The passage of legislation to do research on firearms is encouraging since research and advocacy can move the process, albeit slowly, to help protect children from harm [22].

At the time of publication of this edition, one of the most important advocacy efforts in pediatrics in vaccination support. With a rise in vaccine-preventable illnesses and vaccine hesitancy in the early to mid-2010s, pediatricians became vocal advocates at local and state levels supporting vaccinations for children, specifically those attending public schools. Bills linked to vaccine hesitancy increased during the COVID-19 pandemic [6]. Many physicians partnered with their state and local leaders to advocate for their communities to obtain the COVID-19 vaccine and to advocate against vaccine exemption bills. Dr. Lisa Costello, an Internal Medicine-Pediatrics trained West Virginian pediatrician, partnered with her state and local leaders and the West Virginia Department of Health and Human Resources to advocate for all West Virginians to receive the COVID-19 vaccination [8].

Historically, much of pediatric advocacy included partnering with local, community, state, and federal leaders to promote child health, or writing to news publications about health and development concerns relating to children. During the twenty-first century, with the development and expansion of social media, many pediatricians began using social media platforms to advocate directly to their communities. This social media audience is vast and word travels fast through social media platforms, allowing pediatricians to share their messages quickly beyond their communities, potentially reaching anyone in the world.

Social Media Advocacy

Advocacy in medicine, including pediatrics, has changed as social media sites were launched in the mid-2000s. Social media sites are web-based services that allow individuals to:

1. Construct a public or semipublic profile within a bounded system
2. Articulate a list of other users with whom they share a connection

3. View and traverse their list of connections and those made by others within the system [5]

The most common and widely used sites by the medical community at the time of publication are Facebook®, Twitter®, Instagram™, and, more recently, TikTok®. Some pediatric organizations provide guidance on how to advocate on social media by providing best practice information and practical tips. Medical advocacy on social media has primarily taken two forms:

1. Medical groups and physicians collaborating for patient- or community-centered and legislative advocacy
2. Individual physicians advocating for specific patient- or community-centered initiatives [1]

Child health groups, like the Children's Hospital Association, the AAP, and others, have participated in the collaboration efforts by using their membership to participate in advocacy efforts related to community-centered or legislative advocacy. The AAP's Council on Communication and Media (COCM) used this approach to advocate with communities and lawmakers on behalf of protecting Medicaid and the ACA in 2017. Inspired by then AAP COCM Vice-Chair Dr. Nusheen Ameenuddin, AAP members from across the United States, shared individual videos on Twitter discussing why the ACA was important to the children in their communities. These videos served to inform communities and mobilize other pediatricians to share similar content. The AAP compiled the individual videos into a larger video which the academy and its members used to advocate for continued protection for Medicaid with members of the US House of Representatives and Senate [2].

Individual physicians and/or practices have used their individual or practice social media profiles to advocate on important topics within their communities, including firearm safety and injury prevention, mental healthcare, and vaccines. Pediatricians use social media sites such as Facebook®, Instagram™, Twitter®, and TikTok® to advocate using text, image, and/or video posts. Some posts are educational with information about disease processes, some may have injury prevention information, and others may advocate for injury or disease prevention. Some of these posts have gone "viral," a term used to describe the quick and widely spread or popularized especially by means of social media [18]. Dr. Christina Johns and Dr. Elizabeth Murray, two pediatric emergency medicine physicians, use Dr. Johns' Instagram™ page to discuss current child health issues and weekly updates and information during the COVID-19 pandemic [9].

Many responses to social media advocacy are supportive and bring communities together. However, some responses or comments to certain posts or activities are used to propagate misinformation and have even led to threats against the posters. In response to such events, healthcare providers have banded together to create positive networks and organizations to support one another. One such organization is "Shots Heard Round the World." The group formed in 2017 in response to an attack on a pediatric practices' post related to an educational Facebook® post about the human papillomavirus vaccine. The group aims to educate and defend providers and practices through creating a supporting network. This group and others have helped practices and individuals whose social media posts have been targeted with misinformation and threats [23]. Dr. Nicole Baldwin, a pediatrician and vaccine advocate, turned to Shots Heard Round the World in 2020 when her TikTok® video on childhood vaccinations went viral [16].

Future Advocacy Directions

As pediatrics moves forward, it will continue to be guided by its advocacy-based DNA. The immediate future of pediatric advocacy is focused on:

1. Racial child health equity
2. Transgender and gender-diverse care
3. Climate change
4. Gender equity
5. Child health advocates in government

Racial Child Health Equity

Child health equity is at the forefront of discussion today and racism is a core social determinant of health that drives health inequities. Advocating for community initiatives and collaborating with government- and community-based organizations to help address biases and inequities in the health, justice, and educational systems will help pediatricians advocate for anti-racism in clinical practice and research [25]. Dr. Julie Linton advocates for children from immigrant families and has used her efforts to help legislators understand that immigration status is a social determinant of health [14]. Dr. Rhea Boyd has used her voice to educate her community and colleagues about the challenges children experience due to structural racism [11]. Pediatricians can create culturally safe medical homes by training clinical and office staff in culturally competent care according to national standards for culturally and linguistically appropriate services. Pediatricians can also advocate for racial child health equity by partnering with hospitals and healthcare organizations to conduct internal quality assurance assessments that include analyses of quality of care by race and to initiate improvement protocols as needed to improve health outcomes. Pediatricians can also advocate for federal and local policies that support implicit bias training in schools, including training of educators in culturally competent classroom management to improve disparities in academic outcomes and disproportionate rates of suspension and expulsion among students of color. Pediatricians can support and conduct research examining the impact of policy changes and community-level interventions on reducing the health effects of racism and the impact of perceived and observed experiences of discrimination on child and family health outcomes [25]. Dr. Nia Heard-Garris, the principal investigator at Adversity, Racism, Inequities, Structures (and) Empowerment (ARISE) Health Lab, studies the role adversity and structural inequities play on childhood health [4].

Transgender and Gender-Diverse Care

Caring for the transgender and gender-diverse child is another aspect of child health equity that will be of paramount importance moving forward in the future as the rights of transgender and gender-diverse children are challenged with local and national policies and legislation. Advocacy in this area should include education and partnership with school districts and community organizations to promote acceptance and inclusion of all children. Dr. Deanna Wilson Adkins has advocated to her community against bills designed to ban transgender care [17]. Pediatricians can also advocate within healthcare systems to ensure that electronic health records, billing systems, and clinical research be designed to respect the asserted gender identity of each patient. Lastly, pediatricians can work with health insurances companies to ensure insurance plans offer coverage for healthcare that is specific to the needs of transgender and gender-diverse youth, including coverage for medical, psychological, and, when indicated, surgical gender-affirming interventions [21].

Climate Change

Climate change related to physical, chemical, and ecological changes in the planet uniquely affects children's physical and mental health related to food, water and shelter insecurity, and decreased air quality. Pediatricians can advocate for strategies that improve preparedness for anticipated climate-associated effects, including weather disasters such as floods, droughts, or fires. Pediatricians are also uniquely positioned to advocate for sustainable electricity-generating systems, accessible public and active transportation, plant-based food availability, and green spaces, ultimately improving child and family health. Lastly, pediatricians, like Dr. Ruth Etzel, can advocate for governments to fund research, surveillance, reporting, and tracking of climate-associated health effects [7]. Dr. Etzel's research and knowledge of children's environmental exposures helped her make recommendations to the Office of Children's Health Protection at the US Environmental Protection Agency [15].

Gender Equity

Pediatricians should also work to address the gender leadership inequity within the field. Despite making up over 50% of pediatricians in academic practice and 60% in practice, women make up only 26% of academic pediatric department chairs [24]. All pediatricians, male, female, transgender, non-binary and gender-diverse, should advocate for transparent metrics for pay and promotion (academic and career). These activities should be directed toward academic medical centers and healthcare organizations, professional societies, medical journals, and funding agencies. Additionally, pediatricians should partner with physicians in other medical specialties, like obstetrics/gynecology, internal medicine, and family medicine, to address gender equity in medicine as improving outcomes in all of medicine will also help to improve outcomes in the field of pediatrics. The Executive Leadership in Academic Medicine® (ELAM) program through the Drexel University College of Medicine, under the leadership of pediatrician Dr. Nancy Spector, has helped to develop women to pursue and obtain leadership roles within medicine, including pediatrics [10]. Lastly, pediatricians should partner with the larger national and international gender equity movements to advocate for gender equity for they care for and themselves [24].

Child Health Advocates in Government

2020 was the first year a pediatrician, Dr. Kim Schrier, was elected to the US House of Representatives. In 2021, President Joseph Biden nominated, and the US Senate confirmed, a transgender pediatrician, Dr. Rachel Levine, as Assistant Secretary of Health of the United States. Drs. Schrier and Levine opened the door for more pediatricians and child health advocates in the federal government, helping to establish federal policy. At a local and state level, several pediatricians have run for and been elected to state and local governments. Pediatricians within all levels of government give children and child advocates a voice when policies are discussed, and laws are legislated. Moving forward, pediatricians can improve their advocacy by becoming more involved in their communities and governments, whether it be a local, city, council, or a federal level.

Engaging in Child Health Advocacy

Individual pediatricians and trainees can get involved in child health advocacy by:

- Reading about child health equity challenges at a local, state, federal, and international level
- Reading about local, state, federal, and international child health policy and legislation
- Becoming an active member of state AAP chapter
- Becoming an active member of the APA

References

1. Ameenuddin N. Consider using Twitter to take meaningful action beyond office walls. 2016, November 22. AAP News. https://www.aappublications.org/news/2016/11/22/MasteringMedia112216.
2. American Academy of Pediatrics. Pediatricians Speak Up to Protect Medicaid [Video File]. YouTube. 2017, July 13. https://www.youtube.com/watch?v=1XWdIvP9RBM.
3. American Academy of Pediatrics. The American Academy of Pediatrics 90 Years of Caring for Children 1930–2020. American Academy of Pediatrics. 2020. https://downloads.aap.org/AAP/PDF/9.%20AAP%2090TH%20ANNIVERSARY%20-%20FINAL.pdf.
4. ARISE Health Lab. 2021, June 15. https://arisehealthlab.org/.
5. Boyd DM, Ellison NB. Social network sites: definition, history, and scholarship. J Comput-Mediat Commun. 2007;13(1):210–30. https://doi.org/10.1111/j.1083-6101.2007.00393.x.
6. Burki T. Vaccine misinformation and social media. Lancet Digital Health. 2019;1(6) https://doi.org/10.1016/s2589-7500(19)30136-0.
7. Council on Environmental Health. Global climate change and Children's health. Pediatrics. 2015;136(5):992–7. https://doi.org/10.1542/peds.2015-3232.
8. COVID-19 vaccine. West Virginia Department of Health and Human Resources. 2021, May. https://dhhr.wv.gov/covid-19/pages/vaccine.aspx.
9. Dr. Christina Johns [@deardrchirstina]. n.d.. Posts [Instagram profile]. Instagram. Retrieved August 26, 2021, from https://www.instagram.com/deardrchristina.
10. Drexel University. n.d. Executive Leadership in Academic Medicine. Drexel University College of Medicine. https://drexel.edu/medicine/academics/womens-health-and-leadership/elam/.
11. Frkovich P. Podcast: Big Data, racial bias & a new generation of Organizations: An interview with Dr. Rhea Boyd. All In: Data for Community Health. 2020, June 15. https://www.allindata.org/resources/podcast-big-data-racial-bias-a-new-generation-of-organizations-an-interview-with-dr-rhea-boyd/.
12. Hanna-Attisha M. What the eyes don't see: a story of crisis, resistance, and hope in an American city. One World. 2019.
13. Howell BA, Kristal RB, Whitmire LR, Gentry M, Rabin TL, Rosenbaum J. A systematic review of advocacy curricula in graduate medical education. J Gen Intern Med. 2019;34(11):2592–601. https://doi.org/10.1007/s11606-019-05184-3.
14. Jphmpdirect. North Carolina Pediatrician Julie Linton advocating on behalf of immigrant children. JPHMP Direct. 2017, May 11. https://jphmpdirect.com/2017/05/11/north-carolina-pediatrician-julie-linton-advocating-on-behalf-of-immigrant-children/.
15. Korioth T. Fellows in the News: Dr. Etzel honored for protecting children from environmental chemicals, and more. American Academy of Pediatrics. 2019, January 4. https://www.aappublications.org/news/2019/01/04/fellows010419.
16. Lee BY. How this vaccination video went viral, but resulted in threats against pediatrician. Forbes. 2020, January 20. https://www.forbes.com/sites/brucelee/2020/01/19/how-this-pro-vaccination-video-went-viral-but-resulted-in-threats-against-pediatrician/?sh=1903b785516a.

17. Leslie L. Top transgender doctor warns teen treatment ban could be deadly. 2021, April 9. WRAL.com. https://www.wral.com/top-transgender-doctor-warns-teen-treatment-ban-could-be-deadly/19618762/.
18. Merriam-Webster. Viral. Merriam-Webster. 2021. https://www.merriam-webster.com/dictionary/viral.
19. Miller D. From cover to cover: A look inside AAP blueprint for next administration. AAP News. 2016, October 27. https://www.aappublications.org/news/2016/10/27/Washington102716.
20. Palfrey JS, Hametz P, Grason H, McCaskill QE, Scott G, Chi GW. Educating the next generation of pediatricians in urban health care: the Anne E. Dyson community pediatrics training initiative. Acad Med. 2004;79(12):1184–91. https://doi.org/10.1097/00001888-200412000-00011.
21. Rafferty J, Committee on Psychosocial Aspects of Child and Family Health, Committee on Adolescence, & Section on Lesbian, Gay, Bisexual and Transgender Health and Wellness. Ensuring comprehensive care and support for transgender and gender-diverse children and adolescents. Pediatrics. 2018;142(4) https://doi.org/10.1542/peds.2018-2162
22. Roberts KB, Stein REK, Cheng TL. The academic pediatric association: the first 50 years. Acad Pediatr. 2011;11(3):173–80. https://doi.org/10.1016/j.acap.2011.02.001.
23. Shots Heard Round The World. n.d.. https://www.shotsheard.org/.
24. Spector ND, Asante PA, Marcelin JR, Poorman JA, Larson AR, Salles A, Oxentenko AS, Silver JK. Women in pediatrics: progress, barriers, and opportunities for equity, diversity, and inclusion. Pediatrics. 2019;144(5) https://doi.org/10.1542/peds.2019-2149.
25. Trent M, Dooley DG, Dougé J. The impact of racism on child and adolescent health. Pediatrics. 2019;144(2) https://doi.org/10.1542/peds.2019-1765.

Chapter 14
Supporting the Health and Wellbeing of Women in Pediatrics

Anisha Thaker, Mary Ottolini, and Shilpa J. Patel

> Communities and countries and ultimately the world are only as strong as the health of their women. – Michelle Obama [1]

Background

Wellbeing is an ever-changing aspect of life that varies by individual and requires active awareness, acceptance, and commitment. Women have traditionally taken roles of caregivers, often prioritizing professional and personal responsibilities toward others over their own wellbeing. In order to live fully, women must nurture each of the established dimensions of wellness: physical, social, emotional, intellectual, vocational, environmental, spiritual, and financial [2, 3]. Ignoring or neglecting individual wellbeing can trigger a variety of stressors that often lead to *burnout*, a psychological syndrome characterized by emotional exhaustion, depersonalization, and a reduced sense of personal accomplishment [4].

Healthcare and medical innovations have made significant advances that benefit patients but can also create work environments where physicians are forced to rush

A. Thaker (✉)
University of Massachusetts, Amherst, MA, USA

M. Ottolini
Tufts University School of Medicine and The George W. Hallett MD Chair of Pediatrics, The Barbara Bush Children's Hospital at Maine Medical Center, Portland, ME, USA
e-mail: mottolini@mmc.org

S. J. Patel
Pediatrics at University of Hawaii, John A. Burns School of Medicine, Pediatric Hospitalist at Kapiolani Medical Center for Women & Children, Hawaii Pacific Health, Honolulu, HI, USA
e-mail: shilpa.patel@kapiolani.org

N. D. Spector et al. (eds.), *Women in Pediatrics*,
https://doi.org/10.1007/978-3-030-98222-5_14

patient encounters, are tasked with inefficient clerical work, and which lack ample opportunities for collegiality. The resulting *work compression* undermines the very traits that motivate physicians such as compassion and altruism; serving others devolves into self-sacrificing for others [5]. A recent Medscape report shows that 42% of physicians reported burnout in 2020, with over 70% reporting burnout has a moderate to severe impact on their lives [6]. Women physicians rank significantly higher in all components of empathy which may result in more emotional exhaustion compared to counterparts who are men [7]. The gender differences in burnout – 51% of women physicians reported burnout compared to 36% men physicians – are driven by systemic and societal factors [6].

Physician burnout is a serious problem that can begin as early as medical school. Resident physician burnout is associated with poor work quality, a threefold increase in medical error, and increased guilt about poor patient care [5, 8]. Burnout is also strongly associated with high turnover rates and the cost of recruitment, relocation, onboarding, and ramp-up is approximately two to three times the physician's annual salary [9–17]. Mitigating burnout requires recognition and taking steps to prioritize wellbeing. However, for women physicians especially, physician vulnerability is viewed as a weakness which may negatively impact career opportunities. As a result, burnout is often left unaddressed and unresolved and can result in tragic outcomes.

Each year, more than 1,000,000 patients lose their doctor to suicide, highlighting how physician burnout has ripple effects that devastate broader communities [18]. Physicians commit suicide at rates twice that of the general population and suicide is the cause of the majority of medical student deaths [19]. Women physicians are significantly more likely to commit suicide than men counterparts and twice as more likely as nonphysician women; thus, it is imperative to examine gender-specific differences in the drivers of burnout to tailor systemic interventions for healthier work approaches and environments for women in pediatrics [20].

Drivers of Burnout

Drivers contributing to physician burnout can be grouped into seven dimensions: workload and job demands, efficiency and resources, meaning in work, culture and values, control and flexibility, social support and community at work, and work-life integration [21]. A focused understanding of how women physicians function within these dimensions will promote the ongoing movement toward gender equity.

> *Ann, a pediatric neuro-intensivist, has dedicated her life to providing expert compassionate care to patients with devastating neurologic injury and has single-handedly built the neuro-intensive care unit over the past five years. She learns that the institution will not be hiring a promised additional neuro-intensivist to provide backup call coverage because of other institutional priorities. Ann uncharacteristically raises her voice to argue with her division chief and is referred to human resources and the employee assistance program to "develop skills to cope with job stress."* – Anonymous, 2021

Women like Ann are more likely to endure unsustainable job demands, perhaps because of a need to prove value to the organization, a fear of not being invited to participate in the future, or a concern for patient care. High workload can be a driver of burnout and is compounded by inadequate compensation and/or limited promotion of women pediatricians; nationwide, early- to midcareer women pediatricians earn less than counterparts who are men [22]. Perhaps more disturbing is that as a profession becomes more women-dominated, the overall earnings decrease, with pediatricians being among the lowest paid among all specialties [23, 24]. Insufficient compensation during the COVID-19 pandemic disproportionately burdened primary care physicians and frontline workers, a majority of whom were women [25, 26]. Many women in pediatrics bore the elevated risk and mental stress of contracting COVID-19, the threat of passing the virus to family members, and the uncertainty of needing to take unpaid leave to recover or care for sick relatives, all without proper hazard pay or compensation [27]. Lack of representation of women was evident in addressing pandemic-related issues: despite making up 64% of pediatricians, women hold proportionately few leadership positions [25, 28]. With fewer women at the forefront of institutional, regional, and national policy creation, leadership may inadvertently implement procedures that disadvantage women pediatricians [27]. For example, organizations may implement mandatory "backup" coverage during pandemic surge periods, disregarding conflicts like childcare [27]. Such policies can disproportionately upset career stability or delay advancement opportunities for women [27].

> *Men in my health system do fewer administrative tasks than women, who often volunteer to organize events, take meeting minutes, prepare slide decks, organize holiday gifts for hospital units, etc. These extra tasks, of small and big value, are time consuming and detract from time spent on work that is consistently recognized and valued for promotions or compensation, leaving women doing necessary work that remains unvalued.* –Anonymous, 2021

Burdened with extra clerical work, time-constrained patient visits, and limited scheduling flexibility, 58% of physicians claim bureaucratic tasks are the leading cause of burnout [6]. When established workplace culture and ineffective leadership behaviors hinder employee input in workflow practices and policies, physicians are more likely to feel a deterioration of control, independence, and meaningfulness in work, all significant contributors to burnout [29]. Women in pediatrics report having even less control over workplace decisions than men, which contributes to the gender disparity in high risk for burnout [28]. High work compression environments and electronic communication may also contribute to burnout by displacing spontaneous collegiality and meaningful peer support, especially in the face of challenges like poor patient outcomes, medical errors, and malpractice suits [30–33]. Without *meaningful* peer support, young women physicians are particularly susceptible to burnout since they also often face professional bias and harassment [34–36]. Importantly, while junior women faculty are more likely to receive advice from multiple mentors, men are more likely to be mentored and sponsored by upper level leadership [35, 37, 38]. Fewer women in upper leadership positions means that women mentors often do not have the power to sponsor women mentees [39, 40]. A gender-biased workplace culture may permit discrimination and harassment toward women [36]. It is important to note the "double bind" effect: women physicians with intersectional identities, those who identify with any one or more marginalized community (race, LGBTQ, etc.), face harsher bias and discrimination [41]. A lack of diversity and inclusion among leaders trickles down to impact entering women physicians since they then have less representation and less access to meaningful mentorship and sponsorship; combined with lack of support, this leaves intersectional women more susceptible to burnout [29].

> *When Riya, a pediatric ER physician, was asked by a male boss how it felt to return to work after maternity leave, he was surprised to hear that she was struggling to meet the demands at home with her work schedule, "…but babies are so immobile at 3 months, what do you stay busy with at home?" he had asked.* – Anonymous, 2021

Drivers of burnout are exacerbated for women needing maternity leave or if the return-to-work lifestyle is extremely difficult to reconcile with childcare. Pediatrics is one of the specialties with the highest proportion of women (38%) becoming pregnant during residency [42]. While the American Academy of Pediatrics recommends 6 months to a year of exclusive breastfeeding and extended leave is associated with a longer duration of breastfeeding, residents are only given an average of 6.6 weeks paid maternity leave [43, 44]. Often facing bias regarding taking time to pump and a lack of flexible scheduling or on-site childcare, many women physicians feel forced to ignore the very childcare advice they give to patients [34, 45]. Unintentional gender-biased policies can incorporate maternal discrimination: pregnant women have been expected to perform high-risk tasks involving exposure to communicable diseases that can cause fetal defects or continue to work during preterm labor or while having a miscarriage [45]. These policies often lack support surrounding miscarriage; one-third of 844 physician mothers experienced a miscarriage and only 97 reported being able to take time off to recover [34]. Leadership dominated by men can also be unaware of difficulties women face when leaving their baby and managing with a sleep-deprived schedule. Remarks that minimize the volume and toll of juggling childcare, child-rearing, and return-to-work are commonplace and exemplify one of the many microaggressions faced by women physicians at work that can exacerbate burnout. While 76% of women physicians report experiencing gender-based discrimination in early career, 35.8% of late career women reported facing gender-based discrimination, indicating the chronicity of the problem. Very little research has assessed the effects of aging on women physicians in the workplace. A survey conducted on women in the National Association of Women Executives found that despite 95% of menopausal women reporting physical symptoms and 79% reporting emotional symptoms, few workplace policies address or support women experiencing menopause [46]. Women fearing discrimination and embarrassment may not disclose their symptoms, especially if the topic is viewed as inappropriate [47]. Menopausal symptoms have been associated with emotional exhaustion, an indicator of burnout, and having to discreetly handle these symptoms with low social support at work from superiors and colleagues can be frustrating and isolating for women [48, 49].

> *Although my husband and I shared childcare responsibilities, when there was a 'snow day' we would argue over who had the more critical job responsibilities and I ended up feeling like a neglectful mother. My kids attended rounds a lot...* – Anonymous, 2021

Challenges to work-life integration, a key dimension of physician wellbeing, disproportionately affects women. Inadequate paternity leave policies can result in women bearing more childcare responsibilities. Most residency programs provide little to no paternity leave [43]. The "parenting-load" gender disparity continues throughout child-rearing years. Women are more likely to work fewer hours and take on more household responsibilities and/or hire help in order to mitigate professional burnout, while men are more likely to make time for recreational activities [50]. Reports show that 17% of women physicians claim combining parenthood and work as the most concerning issue, compared to 6% of men [6]. The state of work-life integration worsened for women physicians during the COVID-19 lockdown [50, 51]. With parents working from home and closed childcare facilities, the majority of the parenting, childcare, and home schooling responsibilities fell on women [51]. During the early stages of lockdown, women physicians sacrificed self-care and professional responsibilities in order to allot more time for child and household care compared to counterparts who were men, resulting in a drastic gender difference in research and publications [52, 53]. Women pediatricians often have primary responsibility in the majority of household chores, spend more time on housework, and are less satisfied with their share of household responsibility compared to men [50]. Additionally, women are more likely to be solely responsible for the *cognitive dimension* of household and child-rearing labor: the mental and physical work of anticipating needs, identifying options for filling them, making decisions, and monitoring progress on actions [54]. This "invisible" task is a chronic stressor that makes healthy work-life integration and wellbeing even more untenable for women physicians [21, 55].

Considering the prevalence of stressors across all dimensions of wellbeing and the ramifications associated with decreased physician wellbeing, burnout must be addressed systemically. Although individuals should take certain steps to cultivate protective practices/behaviors, only systemic change will have a strong, long-lasting impact on physician wellbeing [21, 56]. Recent survey data shows that only 35% of physicians have a stress reduction/burnout prevention program at their organization [6]. Of those, 70% claimed they would not be very likely to participate in offered programs as they focus on individual approaches, ignoring necessary policy changes [6]. Re-evaluating policies and leadership can help address the gender disparity in burnout [57]. Many institutions seek to change workplace culture but may lack specific guidance or support on how to create and implement plans. Below are several strategies organizations and individuals can implement to combat burnout and promote wellbeing among women pediatricians.

Solutions

Systemic Solutions

Interventions at the individual, organizational, and structural levels mitigate burnout for physicians [58–62]. Thoughtfully created interventions that target gender-biased policies are needed because organizational drivers of burnout disproportionately affect women [63]. Systemic change within the medical community beginning as early as medical school ensures that future generations of women physicians are less likely to experience burnout.

Medical schools can actively support the wellbeing of trainees by restructuring clinical rotations to incorporate flexibility and by teaching, modeling, and normalizing behaviors that prioritize emotional wellbeing [29]. Schwartz Rounds, for example, show peer support and collegiality can help pediatricians debrief after difficult cases, build comradery among staff, and alleviate work-related distress [57, 64]. Providing instruction, time for reflection, and practice of self-care strategies during medical school and residency training fosters resiliency [29]. Twenty percent of physicians who report burnout have not sought help out of fear of disclosure; eradicating the stigma surrounding therapy and other psychological supports creates an environment where vulnerability is not associated with weakness and doctors feel safe seeking help without damaging career opportunities or advancement [6]. Medical schools can also shift culture by intentionally pursuing inclusivity among leadership to provide mentors and sponsors representative of a diverse body of future physicians.

Postgraduate environments must work harder to change long established systems that perpetuate the gender pay gap and countless disparities at all levels [65]. Re-evaluating organizational leadership effectiveness and inclusivity for employees with intersectional identities can be achieved by using existing research-backed performance, assessment, and training tools that identify and measure a leader's ability to behave inclusively [66]. In order to mitigate implicit bias, organizations must invest in recruiting and developing quality leaders and increase employee diversity in every part of the hiring process [65, 67]. For example, many search committees initially rely on personal networks when considering candidates, which limits variety, especially if leadership is dominated by men [65]. By working to hire more women leaders, organizations can build a reputation of being fair employers and will be more likely to attract women candidates [65]. Making résumés gender-blind by removing personal information can help diminish hiring bias against women [65]. Organizations can make changes to how employees are integrated and developed within the practice, how performance is assessed, and how compensation and promotions are managed to ensure gender bias and discrimination are not factors that hold women employees back, contribute to professional burnout, or prevent retention of quality physicians [65].

Practices that provide more autonomy, regularly ask for and implement physician input, provide clear structure for large care teams, and create opportunities to reshape working conditions by embedding long-term flexibility can help diminish burnout and increase retention of strong employees [67]. Previously, professional success often required employees to work long hours, overextend themselves, and compete heavily in order to be promoted and climb the corporate ladder, which came at the cost of personal wellbeing and healthy work-life integration [68]. Now, with mothers being the primary earners or co-earners in almost two-thirds of American families, organizations need to meet this fundamental shift with a new outlook on career performance and advancement for both women and men [68, 69]. Long-term flexibility involves an organizational shift from the traditional corporate ladder model to a nuanced *corporate lattice* model [68]. While the traditional hierarchy was forged by a singular path upward, assumed the needs of employees remained constant over time, and was more conducive to a traditional family structure where men had to prioritize work over life, the corporate lattice model allows for multiple paths upward where employees have the option to move fast, to move slow, or change directions [68]. In this continuously evolving matrix, the organization adjusts as the needs of employees change over the course of their career, which allows employees to maintain healthier work-life integration and can help diminish burnout [21, 68]. The corporate lattice model also fosters loyalty both for employers and employees, which can help reduce turnover rates and lower the costs of continuous recruitment, onboarding, and starter packages [68]. An example of a corporate lattice model is the *mass career customization* (MCC) framework, which encompasses four dimensions: pace of career progression, workload, location/schedule for work, and job role [68]. Figures 14.1 and 14.2 depict an adapted MCC framework, which follows the career of a physician over several stages of life, showing how the four dimensions can ebb and flow to allow for employee and organizational success [68]. Leaders who understand the sine wave of mass career customization can support, retain, and promote women into leadership by understanding and implementing flexible policies.

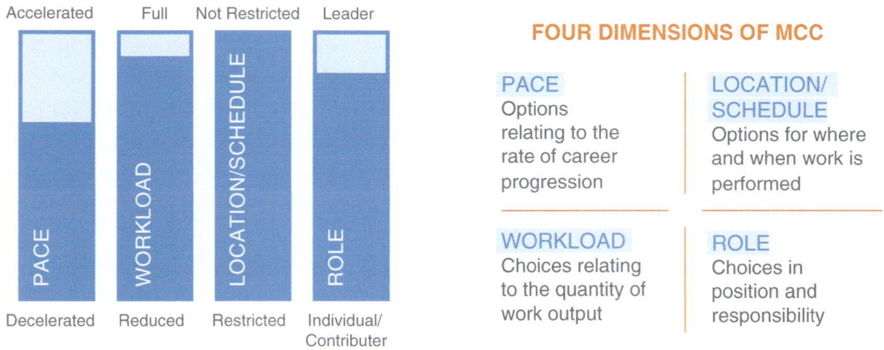

Fig. 14.1 The four dimensions of mass career customization

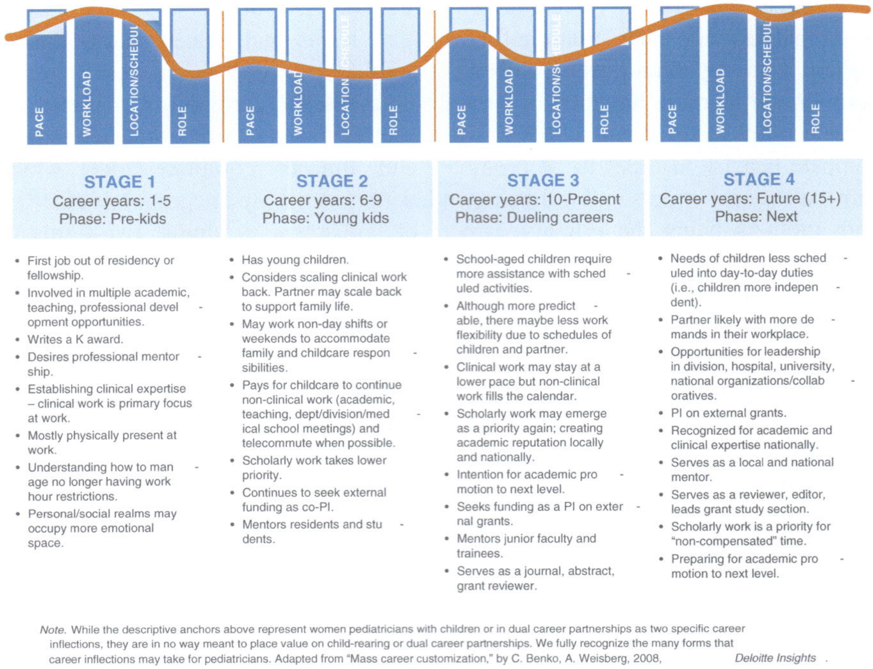

Fig. 14.2 Sine wave for a woman academic pediatrician

A prime example of effectively restructuring workplace policies to incorporate and promote flexibility and autonomy was the Academic Biomedical Career Customization (ABCC) pilot study conducted at Stanford University School of Medicine. Faculty in academic medicine first met with professional coaches to reflect on work-life and work-work challenges and design a plan promoting personal and professional goals that accommodated for any institutional or personal constraints. Team leaders (e.g., division chief) were trained on how to determine a balance between the goals of the team and the goals of the individual faculty member. Leaders were provided guides that listed flexibility and career development policies and examples of how these policies could assist in achievement of personal and professional goals [70]. This first phase of the intervention demonstrated that employee wellbeing is a priority. Leadership training and guidance that incorporates sensitivity toward women, women with intersectional identities, antibias and anti-discrimination training, and inclusive hiring and on-boarding practices prioritizes wellbeing to prevent burnout.

A key segment of the ABCC intervention is a time-banking system which provides choice and flexibility of work schedules, another policy that can alleviate burnout [67, 70]. This time-banking system codified various tasks into "credit" values determined by the team, allowing for customization [70]. Previously, faculty would often "trade favors" and complete work tasks for each other, but with the time-banking system, employees received credits for all extra tasks completed that benefitted the organization or other team members [70]. These credits could be used for support services at home (e.g., free meal for the family or house cleaning) or at work (e.g., hiring grant writing specialists or interview coaches) [70]. Faculty felt encouraged to take on more responsibilities, making it possible for colleagues to decrease workload when needed (e.g., manuscript deadlines or family crisis), thus embedding flexibility in workplace culture and reframing the concept to support both individual and team success [70]. Individual faculty work production could ebb and flow while overall team success remained constant, providing more autonomy and enabling staff to have a healthy sense of control at work, which helps strengthen wellbeing [67, 70].

The time-banking system also fostered collegiality and positive relationships among coworkers because work favors never went unnoticed, ignored, or unreturned; faculty did not feel resentment for extra work completed due to credit compensation [70]. Additionally, recognition and value of their extra work on a shared tracker was associated with positive feelings [70]. In the ABCC pilot, team leaders were able to support faculty wellbeing as participants found stronger purpose at work [21, 67, 70].

A time-banking system could significantly reduce the tension of childcare and work-life integration by applying credits toward support services at home; other colleagues could help share the workload should a family emergency arise. Valuing extra work with a visible, tracked credit system could also help diminish the baseless self-doubt women feel because of the stigma attached to asking for help, thereby reducing drivers of burnout [70, 71]. Some may argue that credits should be translated into salary increments or bonuses, considering 45% of physicians experiencing burnout claim increased compensation would help most to avoid financial stress [6, 70]. However, the ABCC time-banking method works to target solutions supported by the majority of physicians experiencing burnout: 42% voted for a more manageable work and schedule; 39% voted for greater respect from administrators/employers, colleagues, or staff; 35% voted for increased autonomy; and 32% voted for more support staff [6].

Leadership can engage staff through effective professional development, schedule adjustment, and opportunities for peer support. Providing at least 1 hour of protected time for physicians to meet and discuss career-related topics has been shown to increase meaning in work and decrease burnout [61]. These avenues are also opportunities for leadership to promote diversity, equity, and inclusion since women with intersectional identities experience compounded bias and are more likely to experience burnout [41, 72]. Leaders can help women physicians find meaningful mentorship and sponsorship prospects by forming identity-specific peer support groups [28].

Implementing physician input and including physicians in leading efforts to improve workflows contributes to wellbeing [21, 67]. Physicians should identify the roles that best align with their professional interests and purpose. Physicians can engage a coach to assist them in identifying and maximizing the amount of their professional effort that is spent in meaningful roles through inquiry, encouragement, and accountability [67]. This manner of addressing burnout requires both a systemic and an individual culture shift so that physicians feel comfortable being honest about vulnerable areas, working hard through a steep learning curve, and then continuing toward improvement.

A major part of shifting culture and respecting physician feedback will involve addressing childbearing and child-rearing. For pregnant physicians, policies must protect them from completing tasks that can be harmful to their health or the health of the fetus [45]. Long-needed updates on maternity/paternity leave policies must occur. The USA lags behind most developed countries in terms of maternity leave even though research shows that longer paid family leave is positively associated with maternal mental health and breastfeeding [73, 74]. Adequate maternity and paternity leave can help alleviate burnout among women physicians by providing time to heal, emotionally bond with the baby, and share childcare responsibilities with the non-birth parent so that mothers may return to work as balanced and energized as possible. Return-to-work support for physician mothers should entail services and policies providing nearby childcare, adequate breast pumping time without penalty, and flexible scheduling [34]. By making these support systems part of the workplace culture and norms, organizations can eradicate the bias and discrimination many mothers face [34].

Workplace culture can diminish gender bias and support women physicians by normalizing conversation and policy around menopause. Leaders can begin by creating guidance tailored for the organization which incorporates evidence-based research [75]. In environments with men-dominated leadership, it is especially important to increase general awareness about menopause, associated symptoms, and guidance on how to best support women employees during conversations regarding menopause [75, 76]. Flexible scheduling, work from home options and time-banking policies can help provide additional support for women physicians without risking career stability or advancement opportunities [70, 75]. By creating more awareness and normalizing menopause, organizations can aim to further empower and engage women physicians, support employee wellbeing, and avoid the high costs and risks associated with frequent clinician burnout [48, 77].

Bias and discrimination can be eradicated if entire communities work to support women in pediatrics. Physician leaders can teach by example through inclusive hiring practices, meaningful mentorship, and sponsorship. Shifting workplace culture so that physicians feel comfortable being vulnerable and examining their own conscious and subconscious biases will inevitably trickle down to men colleagues, who can practice stronger forms of allyship – a benefit for all [78]. Simultaneously, women in pediatrics need to feel supported by the external community. Often in society, the professional accomplishments of men are celebrated more, while women are more likely to be praised for personal accomplishments like marriage or having children. Both men and women collectively can ask about and celebrate advancements in the careers of women physicians.

Individual Solutions

> *A woman's health is her capital.* – Harriet Beecher Stowe [79]

Seminars and workshops that target individual approaches to diminish burnout and reduce stress and fatigue often frustrate physicians if systemic changes are not being implemented [6]. While institution-level preventative measures like re-evaluating leadership, incorporating flexibility into policies, and creating more diverse and inclusive environments are crucial, implementing these changes can be a slow process marked with red tape and bureaucracy [21, 67]. Therefore, it is important for women physicians to understand how occupational burnout can affect their professional and personal lives. As the traditional caregivers, women are constantly multitasking, both professionally and personally, and overextending themselves for the community at the steep cost of personal wellbeing. By understanding the harsh consequences of ignoring self-care and learning various methods to fight against burnout, women must work to create a personal harmony between the dimensions of wellbeing [2].

Recognizing the neurobiological impacts of burnout can help women identify symptoms and take necessary steps for intervention [67]. In response to chronic occupational stress, women show pronounced partially-reversible structural abnormalities in the prefrontal cortex (PFC), an area of the frontal lobe of the brain that controls high-order reasoning, social cognition, and complex decision-making [67, 80]. Fatigue-induced PFC dysfunction can lead to forgetfulness, reduced motivation, impaired decision-making, unprofessional behavior, decreased empathy and engagement, and impaired communication with patients/coworkers – all characteristics associated with occupational burnout and potential for medical errors [67]. This toxic response in the brain is specifically a result of prolonged *uncontrollable* stress, and as such, a perceived sense of control can protect women from PFC dysfunction [81]. When women physicians are highly stressed, just the awareness of the biochemical changes occurring in the brain can increase perceived control and mitigate PFC impairment [67]. Additionally, this awareness can reduce self-blame, promote a more compassionate view of oneself and others, and provide the opportunity to take necessary steps to care for personal wellbeing [67]. Table 14.1 outlines skills and strategies associated with burnout prevention or mitigation (Table 14.1).

For women to prioritize self-care, recreational activities, and overall wellbeing, women must establish and maintain healthy work-life integration. Women often feel guilty if they do not offer to volunteer for "office housework" or take time for self-care over housework/childcare. It is important to remember the *airplane rule:* "Always put your own oxygen mask on before assisting someone else." Women physicians, and their families, need to accept that self-care is not indulgent or selfish, but necessary. If women do not take the time to refresh and simply have fun, they are more likely to experience the hazardous symptoms of burnout which can have even more damaging repercussions. Women physicians should lean on their social support system and normalize asking for help rather than feeling inadequate that they cannot manage it all alone. In order to find

Table 14.1 Skills and strategies associated with burnout prevention and mitigation

Skills/strategies to develop/implement		Benefits associated with burnout prevention/reduction
Emotional intelligence [82]		Increased sense of control, job satisfaction, patient satisfaction [82], social relationship satisfaction [83]
Self-regulation [82]		
Self-awareness	Naming emotions [67]	
	Identifying when workload is overwhelming [67]	
	Attending physical needs (hunger/sleep) [67]	
	Assertive self-promotion [84]	Increased sense of value/recognition, compensation growth [84]
Recreational activities		Decompressing/refreshing
Mindfulness [67, 85]		Increased activity of PFC in areas that sustain/monitor focus, mitigation of forgetfulness/impaired decision-making associated with PFC dysfunction and burnout, cardiovascular disease prevention [67, 85]
Healthy diet habits		Meet high energy demands of PFC [67, 86]
Exercise		Meet high energy demands of PFC, uplift mood, help with stress coping, enhance sleep quality, CVD prevention [67, 87–89]

support in establishing these boundaries, women can meet with a professional coach to determine individual professional and personal goals and discuss foreseeable constraints in achieving them [67, 70]. Both goal-setting with a coach and maintaining healthy work-life integration can help women physicians have a stronger sense of control, decrease stress, and diminish burnout [21, 61, 67]. Additionally, finding meaningful peer support or actively seeking opportunities to create moments of collegiality can help reduce the isolation and depersonalization associated with burnout [28, 29].

The following anecdote exemplifies several ways that women pediatricians need to be gentle with themselves when work-life integration meets a speed bump.

Mary, a pediatric hospitalist, is resuscitating a baby in respiratory failure when she receives a phone call from her 12-year-old daughter. In the midst of caring for the baby, Mary forgot her daughter's school was on a half day schedule. Her daughter explains that she is in a "stranger's" house using their phone to call to find out when she will be picked up since it is pouring rain. Mary responded, "do the strangers seem nice because I can't get there for a while…"

This story is not meant to condone a mother leaving her child in the rain so she can care for another child, but to exemplify that we must be willing to accept the help of others in times of crisis. Our children will understand that although 99% of the time they come first – sometimes we need to put our patients first as long as we know they are safe. When our children see us accepting help, they also learn to accept help. As women physicians we are blessed to have several wonderful roles in life that we manage to integrate well most of the time. When we juggle a lot of balls, we occasionally drop a few (and they bounce back)! – Anonymous, 2021

Wellbeing of Women in Pediatrics in the Future

We envision a pediatrician mother recommending a career in medicine for her daughter. Times have changed and women physicians experience equity in the workplace and healthy work-life integration. Most importantly, women enjoy lasting meaning and purpose in their work and an authentic, personal harmony with all the dimensions of their wellbeing.

Works Cited

1. Obama M. A passionate, personal case for education [Video]. TED Conferences, Elizabeth G. Anderson School. 2009, April. https://www.ted.com/talks/michelle_obama_a_passionate_personal_case_for_education?language=en.
2. 8 Dimensions of Wellness, (UMD) University of Maryland's Your Guide to Living Well. n.d.. https://umwellness.wordpress.com/8-dimensions-of-wellness/.
3. Stoewen DL. Dimensions of wellness: change your habits, change your life. Can Veterinary J. 2017;58(8):861–2. PubMed.
4. Maslach C, Jackson SE, Leiter MP. Maslach burnout inventory: third edition. In: Evaluating stress: a book of resources. Scarecrow Education; Lanham, MD. 1997. p. 191–218.
5. Mahan JD. Burnout in pediatric residents and physicians: a call to action. Pediatrics. 2017;139(3) https://doi.org/10.1542/peds.2016-4233.
6. Kane L. "Death by 1000 cuts": Medscape National Physician Burnout & suicide report 2021. Medscape. 2021; https://www.medscape.com/slideshow/2021-lifestyle-burnout-6013456
7. Gleichgerrcht E, Decety J. Empathy in clinical practice: how individual dispositions, gender, and experience moderate empathic concern, burnout, and emotional distress in physicians. PLoS One. 2013;8(4):e61526. https://doi.org/10.1371/journal.pone.0061526.
8. Brunsberg KA, Landrigan CP, Garcia BM, Petty CR, Sectish TC, Simpkin AL, Spector ND, Starmer AJ, West DC, Calaman S. Association of Pediatric Resident Physician Depression and Burnout with Harmful Medical Errors on inpatient services. Acad Med. 2019;94(8):1150–6. https://doi.org/10.1097/ACM.0000000000002778.
9. Atkinson W, Misra-Hebert A, Stoller JK. The impact on revenue of physician turnover: an assessment model and experience in a large healthcare center. J Med Pract Manag. 2006;21(6):351–5.
10. Berger JE, Boyle RL Jr. How to avoid the high costs of physician turnover. Med Group Manage J. 1992;39(6):80. 82–84, 86 passim
11. Buchbinder SB, Wilson M, Melick CF, Powe NR. Estimates of costs of primary care physician turnover. Am J Manag Care. 1999;5(11):1431–8.
12. Dewa CS, Loong D, Bonato S, Thanh NX, Jacobs P. How does burnout affect physician productivity? A systematic literature review. BMC Health Serv Res. 2014;14(1):1–10.
13. Misra-Hebert AD, Kay R, Stoller JK. A review of physician turnover: rates, causes, and consequences. Am J Med Qual. 2004;19(2):56–66.
14. Shanafelt T, Sloan J, Satele D, Balch C. Why do surgeons consider leaving practice? J Am Coll Surg. 2011;212(3):421–2.
15. Shanafelt TD, Raymond M, Kosty M, Satele D, Horn L, Pippen J, Chu Q, Chew H, Clark WB, Hanley AE. Satisfaction with work-life balance and the career and retirement plans of US oncologists. J Clin Oncol. 2014;32(11):1127.
16. Williams ES, Konrad TR, Linzer M, McMurray J, Pathman DE, Gerrity M, Schwartz MD, Scheckler WE, Douglas J. Physician, practice, and patient characteristics related to primary

care physician physical and mental health: results from the physician Worklife study. Health Serv Res. 2002;37(1):119.
17. Williams ES, Konrad TR, Scheckler WE, Pathman DE, Linzer M, McMurray JE, Gerrity M, Schwartz M. Understanding physicians: intentions to withdraw from practice: the role of job satisfaction, job stress, mental and physical health. In: Advances in health care management. Emerald Group Publishing Limited; Bingley, UK. 2001.
18. Wible P. 1 million patients lose their doctors to suicide every year. J Med. 2016; https://www.ncnp.org/journal-of-medicine/1782-why-1-million-doctors-kill-themselves-every-year.html
19. Schernhammer E. Taking their own lives—the high rate of physician suicide. N Engl J Med. 2005;352(24):2473–6.
20. Schernhammer ES, Colditz GA. Suicide rates among physicians: a quantitative and gender assessment (meta-analysis). Am J Psychiatr. 2004;161(12):2295–302. https://doi.org/10.1176/appi.ajp.161.12.2295.
21. Shanafelt TD, Noseworthy JH. Executive leadership and physician Well-being: nine organizational strategies to promote engagement and reduce burnout. Mayo Clin Proc. 2017;92(1):129–46. https://doi.org/10.1016/j.mayocp.2016.10.004.
22. Frintner MP, Sisk B, Byrne BJ, Freed GL, Starmer AJ, Olson LM. Gender differences in earnings of early- and midcareer pediatricians. Pediatrics. 2019;144(4):e20183955. https://doi.org/10.1542/peds.2018-3955.
23. Hegewisch A, Williams-Baron E. The Gender wage gap by occupation 2017 and by race and ethnicity. IWPR 2020. 2018, April 29. https://iwpr.org/iwpr-issues/employment-and-earnings/the-gender-wage-gap-by-occupation-2017-and-by-race-and-ethnicity/.
24. Jena AB, Olenski AR, Blumenthal DM. Sex differences in physician salary in US public medical schools. JAMA Intern Med. 2016;176(9):1294–304. https://doi.org/10.1001/jamainternmed.2016.3284.
25. Active Physicians by Sex and Specialty, 2019. n.d. AAMC. Retrieved May 16, 2021, from https://www.aamc.org/data-reports/workforce/interactive-data/active-physicians-sex-and-specialty-2019.
26. Crimi C, Carlucci A. Challenges for the female health-care workers during the COVID-19 pandemic: the need for protection beyond the mask. Pulmonology. 2021;27(1):1–3. PubMed. https://doi.org/10.1016/j.pulmoe.2020.09.004.
27. Jones Y, Durand V, Morton K, Ottolini M, Shaughnessy E, Spector N, O'Toole J. Collateral damage: how COVID-19 is adversely impacting women physicians. J Hosp Med. 2020;15(8):507–9. https://doi.org/10.12788/jhm.3470
28. Spector ND, Asante PA, Marcelin JR, Poorman JA, Larson AR, Salles A, Oxentenko AS, Silver JK. Women in pediatrics: Progress, barriers, and opportunities for equity, diversity, and inclusion. Pediatrics. 2019;144(5):e20192149. https://doi.org/10.1542/peds.2019-2149.
29. Hein C. MMC wellbeing & peer support program. J Maine Med Center. 2021;3(2):17.
30. Hu Y-Y, Fix ML, Hevelone ND, Lipsitz SR, Greenberg CC, Weissman JS, Shapiro J. Physicians' needs in coping with emotional stressors: the case for peer support. Arch Surg. 2012;147(3):212–7.
31. Pratt SD, Jachna BR. Care of the clinician after an adverse event. Int J Obstet Anesth. 2015;24(1):54–63.
32. Shapiro J, Galowitz P. Peer support for clinicians: a programmatic approach. Acad Med. 2016;91(9):1200–4.
33. Wallace JE, Lemaire J. On physician well being—you'll get by with a little help from your friends. Soc Sci Med. 2007;64(12):2565–77.
34. Juengst SB, Royston A, Huang I, Wright B. Family leave and return-to-work experiences of physician mothers. JAMA Netw Open. 2019;2(10):–e1913054. https://doi.org/10.1001/jamanetworkopen.2019.13054.
35. Shakil S, Redberg RF. Gender disparities in sponsorship—how they perpetuate the Glass ceiling. JAMA Intern Med. 2017;177(4):582. https://doi.org/10.1001/jamainternmed.2016.9411.

36. Templeton K, Nilsen KM, Walling A. Issues faced by senior women physicians: a National Survey. J Women's Health. 2020;29(7):980–8. https://doi.org/10.1089/jwh.2019.7910.
37. Ibarra H, Carter NM, Silva C. Why men still get more promotions than women. Harv Bus Rev. 2010;88(9):80–5.
38. Travis EL, Doty L, Helitzer DL. Sponsorship: a path to the academic medicine C-suite for women faculty? Acad Med. 2013;88(10) https://journals.lww.com/academicmedicine/Fulltext/2013/10000/Sponsorship__A_Path_to_the_Academic_Medicine.12.aspx.
39. Ochberg R, Barton G, West A. Women physicians and their mentors. J Am Med Womens Assoc (1972). 1989;44(4):123–6. PubMed
40. Schor NF. The decanal divide: women in decanal roles at U.S. medical schools. Acad Med. 2018;93(2) https://journals.lww.com/academicmedicine/Fulltext/2018/02000/The_Decanal_Divide__Women_in_Decanal_Roles_at_U_S_.30.aspx.
41. Ginther DK, Kahn S, Schaffer WT. Gender, race/ethnicity, and National Institutes of Health R01 research awards: is there evidence of a double bind for women of color? Acad Med. 2016;91(8):1098–107. PubMed. https://doi.org/10.1097/ACM.0000000000001278.
42. Butkus R, Serchen J, Moyer DV, Bornstein SS, Hingle ST. Achieving gender equity in physician compensation and career advancement: a position paper of the American College of Physicians. Ann Intern Med. 2018;168(10):721–3. https://doi.org/10.7326/M17-3438.
43. Magudia K, Bick A, Cohen J, Ng TSC, Weinstein D, Mangurian C, Jagsi R. Childbearing and family leave policies for resident physicians at top training institutions. JAMA. 2018;320(22):2372–4. https://doi.org/10.1001/jama.2018.14414.
44. Pac JE, Bartel AP, Ruhm CJ, Waldfogel J. Paid family leave and breastfeeding: evidence from California. National Bureau of Economic Research Working Paper Series, No. 25784. 2019. https://doi.org/10.3386/w25784.
45. Halley MC, Rustagi AS, Torres JS, Linos E, Plaut V, Mangurian C, Choo E, Linos E. Physician mothers' experience of workplace discrimination: a qualitative analysis. BMJ. 2018;363:k4926. https://doi.org/10.1136/bmj.k4926.
46. Simon JA, Reape KZ. Understanding the menopausal experiences of professional women. Menopause. 2009;16(1) https://journals.lww.com/menopausejournal/Fulltext/2009/16010/Understanding_the_menopausal_experiences_of.14.aspx
47. Hardy C, Griffiths A, Thorne E, Hunter M. Tackling the taboo: talking menopause-related problems at work. Int J Workplace Health Manag. 2019;12(1):28–38. https://doi.org/10.1108/IJWHM-03-2018-0035.
48. Converso D, Viotti S, Sottimano I, Loera B, Molinengo G, Guidetti G. The relationship between menopausal symptoms and burnout. A cross-sectional study among nurses. BMC Womens Health. 2019;19(1):148. https://doi.org/10.1186/s12905-019-0847-6.
49. Reynolds F. Distress and coping with hot flushes at work: implications for counsellors in occupational settings. Couns Psychol Q. 1999;12(4):353–61. https://doi.org/10.1080/09515079908254105.
50. Starmer AJ, Frintner MP, Matos K, Somberg C, Freed G, Byrne BJ. Gender discrepancies related to pediatrician work-life balance and household responsibilities. Pediatrics. 2019;144(4):e20182926. https://doi.org/10.1542/peds.2018-2926.
51. Randell KA, Patel AK, Talib HJ. Parenting pressures among academic pediatricians during the COVID-19 pandemic. Pediatrics. 2021;147(4):e2020033159. https://doi.org/10.1542/peds.2020-033159.
52. Miller KA, Mannix R, Schmitz G, Monuteaux MC, Lee LK. Impact of COVID-19 on professional and personal responsibilities of Massachusetts physicians. Am J Emerg Med. 2020;38(11):2365–7. https://doi.org/10.1016/j.ajem.2020.08.051.
53. Vincent-Lamarre P, Sugimoto CR, Lariviere V. The decline of women's research production during the coronavirus pandemic. Nature Index. 2020;
54. Daminger A. The cognitive dimension of household labor. Am Sociol Rev. 2019;84(4):609–33. https://doi.org/10.1177/0003122419859007.

55. Ciciolla L, Luthar SS. Invisible household labor and ramifications for adjustment: mothers as captains of households. Sex Roles. 2019;81(7):467–86. https://doi.org/10.1007/s11199-018-1001-x.
56. Scheurer D, McKean S, Miller J, Wetterneck T. U.S. physician satisfaction: a systematic review. J Hosp Med. 2009;4(9):560–8. https://doi.org/10.1002/jhm.496.
57. Kase SM, Gribben JL, Waldman ED, Weintraub AS. A pilot study exploring interventions for physician distress in pediatric subspecialists. Pediatr Res. 2020;88(3):398–403. https://doi.org/10.1038/s41390-020-0805-x.
58. Linzer M, Poplau S, Grossman E, Varkey A, Yale S, Williams E, Hicks L, Brown RL, Wallock J, Kohnhorst D. A cluster randomized trial of interventions to improve work conditions and clinician burnout in primary care: results from the healthy work place (HWP) study. J Gen Intern Med. 2015;30(8):1105–11.
59. Panagioti M, Panagopoulou E, Bower P, Lewith G, Kontopantelis E, Chew-Graham C, Dawson S, Van Marwijk H, Geraghty K, Esmail A. Controlled interventions to reduce burnout in physicians: a systematic review and meta-analysis. JAMA Intern Med. 2017;177(2):195–205.
60. West CP, Dyrbye LN, Erwin PJ, Shanafelt TD. Interventions to prevent and reduce physician burnout: a systematic review and meta-analysis. Lancet. 2016;388(10057):2272–81.
61. West CP, Dyrbye LN, Rabatin JT, Call TG, Davidson JH, Multari A, Romanski SA, Hellyer JMH, Sloan JA, Shanafelt TD. Intervention to promote physician Well-being, job satisfaction, and professionalism: a randomized clinical trial. JAMA Intern Med. 2014;174(4):527–33. https://doi.org/10.1001/jamainternmed.2013.14387.
62. West CP, Dyrbye LN, Shanafelt TD. Physician burnout: contributors, consequences and solutions. J Intern Med. 2018;283(6):516–29.
63. Eden AR, Jabbarpour Y, Morgan ZJ, Dai M, Coffman M, Bazemore A. Gender differences in personal and organizational mechanisms to address burnout among family physicians. J Am Board Family Med. 2020;33(3):446. https://doi.org/10.3122/jabfm.2020.03.190344.
64. Adamson K, Sengsavang S, Myers-Halbig S, Searl N. Developing a compassionate culture within pediatric rehabilitation: does the Schwartz rounds™ support both clinical and nonclinical hospital workers in managing their work experiences? Qual Health Res. 2018;28(9):1406–20. https://doi.org/10.1177/1049732318768239.
65. Ammerman C, Groysberg B. How to close the gender pay gap. Harvard Business Review. 2021, June. https://hbr.org/2021/05/how-to-close-the-gender-gap.
66. Rahim-Dillard S. How inclusive is your leadership? Harvard Business Review. 2021, April 19.
67. Arnsten AFT, Shanafelt T. Physician distress and burnout: the neurobiological perspective. Mayo Clin Proc. 2021;96(3):763–9. https://doi.org/10.1016/j.mayocp.2020.12.027.
68. Benko C, Weisberg A.. Mass Career Customization. Deloitte Insights. 2008, August 2. https://www2.deloitte.com/us/en/insights/deloitte-review/issue-3/mass-career-customization-building-the-corporate-lattice-organization.html.
69. Shriver M, Boushey H, O'Leary A. The Shriver report: a woman's nation changes everything. Center for American Progress. 2009, October 16.
70. Fassiotto M, Simard C, Sandborg C, Valantine H, Raymond J. An integrated career coaching and time-banking system promoting flexibility, wellness, and success: a pilot program at Stanford University School of Medicine. Acad Med. 2018;93(6):881–7. PubMed. https://doi.org/10.1097/ACM.0000000000002121
71. Tulshyan R, Burey J-A. Stop telling women they have imposter syndrome. Harvard Business Review. 2021, February 11.
72. Nunez-Smith M, Pilgrim N, Wynia M, Desai MM, Jones BA, Bright C, Krumholz HM, Bradley EH. Race/ethnicity and workplace discrimination: results of a National Survey of physicians. J Gen Intern Med. 2009;24(11):1198. https://doi.org/10.1007/s11606-009-1103-9.
73. Hamad R, Modrek S, White JS. Paid family leave effects on breastfeeding: a quasi-experimental study of US policies. Am J Public Health. 2019;109(1):164–6. https://doi.org/10.2105/AJPH.2018.304693.

74. Staehelin K, Bertea PC, Stutz EZ. Length of maternity leave and health of mother and child – a review. Int J Public Health. 2007;52(4):202–9. https://doi.org/10.1007/s00038-007-5122-1.
75. Hardy C. Menopause and the workplace guidance: what to consider. Post Reproduct Health. 2020;26(1):43–5. https://doi.org/10.1177/2053369119873257.
76. Hardy C, Griffiths A, Hunter MS. What do working menopausal women want? A qualitative investigation into women's perspectives on employer and line manager support. Maturitas. 2017;101:37–41. https://doi.org/10.1016/j.maturitas.2017.04.011.
77. Smeur E. The effect of menopausal complaints on burnout. n.d.
78. Johnson WB, Smith DG. Male Allyship is About Paying Attention. Harvard Business Review. 2021, February 10. https://hbr.org/2021/02/male-allyship-is-about-paying-attention.
79. Stowe HB. Household Papers and Stories. The Riverside Press, Cambridge. n.d. Retrieved November 9, 2021, from https://www.gutenberg.org/files/31217/31217-h/31217-h.htm.
80. Savic I, Perski A, Osika W. MRI shows that exhaustion syndrome due to chronic occupational stress is associated with partially reversible cerebral changes. Cereb Cortex. 2018;28(3):894–906. https://doi.org/10.1093/cercor/bhw413.
81. Glass DC, Reim B, Singer JE. Behavioral consequences of adaptation to controllable and uncontrollable noise. J Exp Soc Psychol. 1971;7(2):244–57. https://doi.org/10.1016/0022-1031(71)90070-9.
82. Weng H-C, Hung C-M, Liu Y-T, Cheng Y-J, Yen C-Y, Chang C-C, Huang C-K. Associations between emotional intelligence and doctor burnout, job satisfaction and patient satisfaction. Med Educ. 2011;45(8):835–42.
83. Lopes PN, Salovey P, Straus R. Emotional intelligence, personality, and the perceived quality of social relationships. Personal Individ Differ. 2003;35(3):641–58.
84. Carter NM, Silva C. The myth of the ideal worker: does doing all the right things really get women ahead? New York: Catalyst; 2011.
85. Tomasino B, Fabbro F. Increases in the right dorsolateral prefrontal cortex and decreases the rostral prefrontal cortex activation after-8 weeks of focused attention based mindfulness meditation. Brain Cogn. 2016;102:46–54. https://doi.org/10.1016/j.bandc.2015.12.004.
86. Engelfriet P, Hoekstra J, Hoogenveen R, Büchner F, van Rossum C, Verschuren M. Food and vessels: the importance of a healthy diet to prevent cardiovascular disease. Eur J Cardiovasc Prev Rehabil. 2010;17(1):50–5. https://doi.org/10.1097/HJR.0b013e32832f3a76.
87. Edenfield TM, Blumenthal JA. Exercise and stress reduction. In: The handbook of stress science: biology, psychology, and health. Springer Publishing Company; New York. 2011. p. 301–19.
88. Karr S. Avoiding physician burnout through physical, emotional, and spiritual energy. Curr Opin Cardiol. 2019;34(1) https://journals.lww.com/co-cardiology/Fulltext/2019/01000/Avoiding_physician_burnout_through_physical.15.aspx
89. Tian D, Meng J. Exercise for prevention and relief of cardiovascular disease: prognoses, mechanisms, and approaches. Oxidative Med Cell Longev. 2019;2019:3756750. https://doi.org/10.1155/2019/3756750.

Chapter 15
Conclusion: Women in Pediatrics

Jennifer K. O'Toole, Barbara Overholser, and Nancy D. Spector

Conclusion

The contributions of women practicing in the specialty of pediatrics have been tremendous over the past century. Women have been pivotal in the specialty's clinical, research, educational, and advocacy efforts and have helped shape the course of the specialty. Women are still avidly entering the specialty and continue to advocate for the health and well-being of all children, all while balancing roles as mothers, caregivers, partners, mentors, and sponsors. Women in pediatrics have been central in building national organizations and research collaboratives that have helped advance child health at the local, national, and global level. Despite all these fundamental contributions, the well-being and success of women in pediatrics is at risk. Faced with systemic bias, discrimination, harassment, and inequity in the setting of the world's most dangerous pandemic in the past century, women may opt to not enter or leave the specialty or the practice of medicine all together. Therefore, the time is now to put forth interventions, policies, and practices that support and elevate

J. K. O'Toole (✉)
Internal Medicine-Pediatrics Residency Program, Departments of Internal Medicine and Pediatrics, University of Cincinnati College of Medicine, Cincinnati Children's Hospital Medical Center, Cincinnati, OH, USA
e-mail: jennifer.otoole@cchmc.org

B. Overholser
Drexel University College of Medicine, Executive Leadership in Academic Medicine® (ELAM), Philadelphia, PA, USA
e-mail: Bro29@drexel.edu

N. D. Spector
Executive Leadership in Academic Medicine® (ELAM), Office of Faculty, Drexel University College of Medicine, Philadelphia, PA, USA
e-mail: Nds24@drexel.edu

N. D. Spector et al. (eds.), *Women in Pediatrics*,
https://doi.org/10.1007/978-3-030-98222-5_15

women in the field and ensure future generations every opportunity for success in their careers.

As a specialty that prides itself on promoting prevention, cultivating long-standing relationships, and supporting the health and well-being of children and their families, there is no better group to lead the way in charting a new course for women in medicine than pediatrics. However, this cannot be accomplished solely by women in the field. We need men to step up, acknowledge the bias and discrimination women face, and use their power, influence, and position to help create a more equitable workplace for women in the specialty. Our hospitals and professional organizations must also become critical change agents in supporting a cycle of improvement and systemic culture and policy change to support and equitably value women in the field.

Women in pediatrics stand on the auspicious shoulders of women like Drs. Jacobi, Elliot, and Epps (discussed in Chap. 1) who paved the way for all women currently practicing in the field. However, progress is still moving at glacial speed. We need *rapid acceleration*. Now is the time to support the disruption of structures that prevent women from advancing and thriving. We need leaders at all levels and of all gender identities that are invested in accelerating diversity, equity, and inclusion efforts. It is our sincere wish that when another group of authors seeks to write the next book about women in pediatrics in 10, 20, or 50 years, they will tell a very different story – a story in which discrimination, bias, and inequity are eliminated and the story of a workplace where women are truly valued, supported, and elevated and have access to a fully equitable workplace. These changes are not just important for women in the field, but also to ensure optimal healthcare and well-being of the most vulnerable population in the world – our children.

Index

N. D. Spector et al. (eds.), *Women in Pediatrics*,
https://doi.org/10.1007/978-3-030-98222-5

MIX
Papier aus verantwortungsvollen Quellen
Paper from responsible sources
FSC® C105338

If you have any concerns about our products,
you can contact us on
ProductSafety@springernature.com

In case Publisher is established outside the EU,
the EU authorized representative is:
Springer Nature Customer Service Center GmbH
Europaplatz 3, 69115 Heidelberg, Germany

Printed by Libri Plureos GmbH
in Hamburg, Germany